CHILD GUIDANCE IN BRITAIN, 1918–1955:
THE DANGEROUS AGE OF CHILDHOOD

Studies for the Society for the Social History of Medicine

Series Editors: David Cantor
                    Keir Waddington

Titles in this Series

CHILD GUIDANCE IN BRITAIN, 1918–1955:
THE DANGEROUS AGE OF CHILDHOOD

BY

John Stewart

Routledge
Taylor & Francis Group

LONDON AND NEW YORK

First published 2013 by Pickering & Chatto (Publishers) Limited

Published 2016 by Routledge
2 Park Square, Milton Park, Abingdon, Oxfordshire OX14 4RN
711 Third Avenue, New York, NY 10017, USA

First issued in paperback 2015

Routledge is an imprint of the Taylor & Francis Group, an informa business

BRITISH LIBRARY CATALOGUING IN PUBLICATION DATA

Stewart, John, author.
Child guidance in Britain, 1918–1955: the dangerous age of childhood. –
(Studies for the Society for the Social History of Medicine)
1. Child welfare – Great Britain – History – 20th century. 2. Child development – Great Britain– History– 20th century.
I. Title II. Series
362.7'0941'09041-dc23

ISBN-13: 978-1-138-66231-5 (pbk)
ISBN-13: 978-1-8489-3429-0 (hbk)

Typeset by Pickering & Chatto (Publishers) Limited

CONTENTS

ACKNOWLEDGEMENTS

This book has been a long time in the making and I have incurred many debts. I would like to thank the Rockefeller Archive Center, New York, the Wellcome Trust and the Royal Society of Edinburgh for awards which allowed me to visit key archives and libraries and to have time away from teaching and administrative duties to research and write. Visiting Fellowships at the University of Bergen, the University of Trier, the University of Southern Denmark and the University of Auckland likewise afforded me time and space as well as intellectual stimulation. I am also grateful for the support of colleagues at the Centre for the Social History of Health and Healthcare, Glasgow, which I was lucky enough to lead between 2007 and 2012. Among those who have helped my understanding of child guidance, either through discussions, comments on papers or through reading and critiquing drafts are Astri Andresen, Linda Bryder, Hera Cook, Janet Greenlees, John Hall, Sarah Hayes, Harry Hendrick, Kathleen Jones, Alysa Levene, Vicky Long, Kari Ludvigsen, Linda McKie, Mary-Clare Martin, Jim Mills, Chris Nottingham, Heather Munro Prescott, Matthew Smith, Sister Gail Taylor, Mathew Thomson and John Welshman. Two anonymous referees provided constructive feedback. Finally, I would like to thank the series editor, Keir Waddington, and Pickering & Chatto staff for their help and support.

LIST OF TABLES

LIST OF ABBREVIATIONS

APSW	Association of Psychiatric Social Workers
BMA	British Medical Association
BMJ	*British Medical Journal*
BPS	British Psychological Society
CGC	Child Guidance Council
CMO	Chief Medical Officer
EIS	Educational Institute of Scotland
GP	General Practitioner
LCC	London County Council
LEA	Local Education Authority
LSE	London School of Economics
MOH	Medical Officer of Health
NAMH	National Association for Mental Health
NHS	National Health Service
NUT	National Union of Teachers
PSW	Psychiatric Social Worker
SAMW	Scottish Association for Mental Welfare
SED	Scottish Education Department
SMO	School Medical Officer

INTRODUCTION: 'AN ENIGMA TO THEIR PARENTS'

In 1929 two psychiatrists associated with the Jewish Child Guidance Clinic in the East End of London, Noel Burke and Emanuel Miller, published an article in the professional outlet *British Journal of Medical Psychology*. Their topic was 'child mental hygiene', an issue which, they claimed, had only recently been subject to a 'more scientific attitude ... coupled to philanthropy'.[1] The following year Miller was again in print, this time in the recently founded popular journal *Mother and Child*. This article was entitled 'The Difficult Child' and in his opening remarks Miller commented that 'with the growth of civilization to the complex form that it has assumed today' children could no longer pass easily from childhood to adolescence to maturity as had previously been the case in 'primitive societies'. Indeed it had to be recognized that the pressures of contemporary life had 'brought about strains and tensions and disruptive tendencies which probably did not exist before'.[2]

Around a year later, in autumn 1931, the Notre Dame Child Guidance Clinic opened in Glasgow, an event described by the local Catholic newspaper. Central to the composition of the clinic, it was suggested, was a team consisting of a psychiatrist, a psychologist and a psychiatric social worker (PSW). The clinic's aim was not to deal with children who had 'definite organic disease, mental defect, or epilepsy'. Rather, its object was the 'study and treatment of children who, though given average home and school conditions, remain an enigma to their parents'.[3]

Some six years later Douglas MacCalman, a psychiatrist who had worked at Notre Dame before becoming General Secretary of the Child Guidance Council (CGC) in London, addressed the Royal Institute of Public Health and Hygiene on the subject of 'The Management of the Difficult Child'. Part of his argument was that while all the causes of a child's emotional and psychological difficulties were as yet unknown, what had been ascertained was that 'parent–child relationships play a huge part in the production of nervous and behaviour disorders'. Was it a 'visionary dream', he asked, that 'a vast system of parent education could be organized?'[4] In 1955, meanwhile, an official committee investigating 'maladjusted children' noted that while 'maladjustment' was a term used in Britain since the 1920s it had only been widely adopted since the Second World War. Although the 'worst effects' of maladjustment were seen among adults, nonetheless it had come 'to be regarded as a problem of childhood'.[5]

This book addresses the issues raised by these extracts. It does so by analysing and describing the origins and development of child guidance and what it sought to achieve. In so doing it engages with concepts such as 'maladjustment' and 'normalcy' in children, why the former was seen as a threat to the child, its family and the wider society and the ways in which 'normalcy' could be regained. Child guidance was, though, highly contested. There were, for instance, disagreements between psychiatrists and psychologists over the causes of maladjustment and, thereby, over how to deal with emotional and psychological problems in childhood. More broadly, this book places child guidance in its wider context, asking why, for example, it saw itself as 'scientific' and what precisely were the problems deriving from 'modernity' or, as Miller put it in 'The Difficult Child', 'civilization in the complex form that it has assumed today'.

In this historical analysis we will encounter individuals such as John Bowlby, William Moodie and Douglas MacCalman, all prominent psychiatrists heavily involved in the medical side of child guidance; the pre-eminent psychologist of the first part of the century, Cyril Burt, and professional supporters such as James Drever and William Boyd; the psychiatric social workers Sybil Clement Brown and Robina Addis, both pioneers of this new profession; social reformers Anne St Loe Strachey and Evelyn Fox; and Mildred Scoville, a key official of the American philanthropic body the Commonwealth Fund of New York. The period covered is from the end of the First World War to the mid-1950s. Child guidance was established in Britain in the late 1920s, grew in scope and ambition in the 1930s and was statutorily recognized as the Second World War came to an end, thus embedding it as part of the emerging welfare state. The chronological end point is the mid-1950s, the period of the official report on the maladjusted child and the reaction to it. At first glance this trajectory appears a triumph for a particular version of child guidance – what we shall come to call the American, or medical, model – in which psychiatric medicine predominated.

However, in reality the situation was more complicated. As noted, throughout child guidance's history there were tensions between psychiatrists and psychologists. The way in which child guidance was situated in the welfare state appeared to favour the latter at the expense of the former, thereby undermining the strictly 'medical' approach which its early proponents sought. There were, moreover, problems involved in ascertaining what constituted normalcy in emotional and psychological health and in assessing the efficacy of diagnosis and treatment. Equally, other forms of child psychiatry were sceptical about the child guidance approach. Little wonder, then, that critical outsiders such as the epidemiologist Jerry Morris argued, in the late 1950s, that child guidance was 'little more than an act of faith'.[6] This was a serious charge given Morris's rising professional status and his role in promoting social medicine. The latter was a branch of the discipline to which, as we shall see in chapter 7, some child guidance supporters aspired. With the benefit of historical hindsight Morris's might be seen to be a harsh but not unreasonable judgement and will be returned to in the concluding chapter.

Nonetheless, British child guidance in the period under analysis was an important expansion of the range and nature of child mental health and welfare services as well as having broader implications with respect to, for example, how child–parent relationships were viewed and family policy and social work practice constructed and delivered. The historiography of child guidance is discussed more fully later in this chapter but it is worth noting here the observations of one historian and two social scientists. Harry Hendrick remarks that by the interwar period the emphasis in child welfare and medicine had changed from a primary concern with 'bodies' to a greater concern with 'minds' and that child guidance was a central component of this refocusing. As Hendrick further notes, child guidance also influenced other aspects of welfare policy, not least the crucial 1948 Children Act. It had, he suggests, stressed the 'importance of childhood as a formative period and the necessity for it to have a stable environment' and this in turn fed into the new kind of relationship between the state and the family which the 1948 Act embodied.[7]

Nikolas Rose argues that the child guidance clinic and the knowledge it generated 'provided the basis for a concerted attempt to disseminate the norms for happy families and contented children which the new psychology had made possible'. Child guidance thus, as Rose further and famously remarked, established a 'systematization of the field of childhood pathology' – childhood had itself, in other words, come to be seen as inherently problematic.[8] More broadly, the twentieth century saw thereby

> the discovery of all those minor mental troubles of children, which became understood in terms of maladjustment or childhood neuroses, which, if left untreated, might develop into frank mental illness – the field of child guidance clinics and later of child psychiatry.

Revealingly, Rose contrasts the 'mild neuroses of child guidance – bed wetting, night terrors, separation anxiety, fear of the dark and the like' with present-day perceptions of the depth and extent of child and adolescent mental ill-health.[9] The view of childhood as a pathological condition has, by this account, deepened and widened even further.

David Armstrong, charting the rise of 'surveillance medicine', points to the child as the 'first target' of the twentieth-century shift towards the 'observation of seemingly healthy populations' and the 'problematisation of the normal'. As he further puts it, the child's 'psychological growth was construed as inherently problematic, precariously normal'. Consequently the child who was nervous, delicate, eneuretic, neuropathic, maladjusted, difficult, neurotic, over-sensitive, unstable or solitary 'emerged as a new way of seeing a potentially hazardous normal childhood'.[10] As we shall see, it was just such children with whom child guidance sought to deal. More generally one very obvious characteristic of child guidance was its employment of medicalized language – the child patient was seen at a clinic where symptoms were diagnosed in order to find the underlying aetiology which in turn led to appropriate treatment.

The analyses of Hendrick, Rose and Armstrong are here taken as important interpretative starting points. In particular, it will be argued that child guidance was seen not simply as an end in itself. Rather, it was an important constituent of a wider concern for political and social stability as well as a mechanism for promoting the aspirations of the professions involved. Underpinning this volume, moreover, is the idea, shared with the three authors just cited, that childhood is not simply a biological construct but is also socially and historically shaped. So, for example, what is considered 'abnormal' behaviour in one historical era may be perfectly acceptable in another. By the same token, though, if childhood of itself is seen as inherently problematic then the behaviours may change but the underlying pathology remains. The remainder of this book seeks to put more empirical flesh on these conceptual bones than has previously been the case through the utilization of, for instance, previously unexplored records from a wide range of individual clinics.

The Growth and Impact of Child Guidance

As a crude indicator of the development of British child guidance, in 1927 Burke and Miller's clinic was the only institution describing itself as concerned with child guidance. Significantly, given the subsequent development of the movement, 1927 also saw the formation of the Child Guidance Council while in 1929 a second clinic opened in London. Crucially, both the Council and the London Child Guidance Clinic (the London Clinic) were financially supported by the Commonwealth Fund of New York, the body central to the founding and expansion of child guidance in both the United States and Great Britain.[11] As a post-war report on social workers in the mental health services remarked, British child guidance 'drew its inspiration from the pioneer work of the Commonwealth Fund' and it was 'difficult to see how either child guidance or psychiatric social work could have started without their support'.[12] This was indeed the case, although the question of the extent of American influence on British child guidance theory and practice is rather more problematic.

By the outbreak of the Second World War there were over sixty British clinics. When combined with the lessons drawn from wartime evacuation surveys – in which child guidance workers played a notable role – this process of expansion led to child guidance being embedded in the post-war welfare state. This came about primarily as a result of the Education Acts of the mid-1940s which empowered local authorities to provide free child guidance services and it is at this point that we find the first official definition of the maladjusted child. In certain respects this was an extension of the Board of Education's ruling in 1935 that local authorities could financially support clinics in their area and which thus constituted the start of a shift away from voluntary to statutory provision. The position of child guidance was further reinforced by the passage of the National Health Service Acts in the mid-1940s. In this climate the number of clinics continued to rise, with the Committee on Maladjusted Children (the Underwood Committee) reporting in 1955 the existence of some 300 such institutions of in England and Wales.[13]

Historians and Child Guidance

Despite its significance child guidance remains under-explored by historians of childhood and child welfare in Britain.[14] Its importance is, as we have seen, widely acknowledged in general terms. In addition to Hendrick, Rose and Armstrong, scholars such as Adrian Wooldridge have recognized the role of child guidance in shaping modern childhood and child welfare services.[15] Mathew Thomson, in a brief discussion of interwar child guidance, is rather more sceptical of its part in psychologizing children, but this of itself suggests the need for a much more systematic attempt to discuss its scale and impact.[16]

There are three, partial, exceptions to this relative historiographical neglect. The first comes from Deborah Thom.[17] Admirable as her essay is, it tells only part of the story, unsurprisingly given the limitations of space. Thom has virtually nothing to say about child guidance outside London and only takes the story down to 1939. Second, we have the chapter by Sarah Hayes which gives fresh insights into the concept of maladjustment and draws in places on child guidance material.[18] Again, though, the latter is only part of her story and she too operates under space constraints. The third exception comes in the form of accounts of child guidance's development from professional participants. These include the history by the psychologist Olive Sampson and that by Robina Addis and John Bowlby's later recollections.[19] Such writings are important, giving as they do a view from the 'inside'. Nonetheless, they tend to take a particular professional standpoint and generally neglect the broader context. Consequently their use for historians is principally as further primary sources.

In short, there has been no systematic attempt to date to provide a comprehensive history of child guidance in Britain from its inception through to the mid-1950s. Child guidance thus exemplifies the argument made by Roger Cooter that in Britain we have only a limited body of writing on children's medical welfare.[20] This scholarly neglect is thrown into even sharper focus when we consider the situation in the United States. Here scholars have exhaustively documented and analysed the child guidance movement. As one such scholar, Kathleen W. Jones, remarks, its history is a 'labyrinthine tale of combinations and confrontations – professional and professional, medicine and social reform, expert and family, parent and child – and the age, class, and gender tensions of the early twentieth century that gave meaning to these connections.'[21]

These observations hold true for the British experience and the aim of the present volume is to provide the sort of scholarly account that Jones and others have provided for the United States. The present author's own previous work is brought to bear and in some cases amended or qualified.

Child Guidance Described

Our analysis is developed more fully in subsequent chapters, but to give some idea of what constituted child guidance, this section expands on the introductory points to give a broad outline of what was involved. Child guidance was initially part of a broader international movement seeking to promote 'mental hygiene' and which in so doing drew upon the so-called 'new psychology'. The campaign for mental hygiene, at its height in the interwar era, saw itself as adopting a preventive medicine approach to mental health issues.[22] As the Scottish psychiatrist and later proponent of child guidance D. K. Henderson told colleagues in 1923, 'this topic of mental hygiene is a live one, one that is engrossing the attention of all of us, whether or not we are psychiatrists, who are interested in the problems of preventive medicine.'[23]

Childhood was particularly important to mental hygiene since, it was believed, mental illness in adults often derived from childhood experience. More than this, though, childhood was the best time to treat such incipient problems as the mind was, at this stage, especially impressionable – 'plastic' in contemporary parlance – and maladjustment had not had time to become deeply entrenched. All this informed the preventive medicine approach. Letitia Fairfield was School Medical Officer (SMO) for the London County Council (LCC). In 1929 she addressed a meeting of the National Council for Mental Hygiene on child guidance and mental hygiene. Modern criminology and modern psychology, although starting from different intellectual positions, had nonetheless 'united in demonstrating the importance of childish habit-formation and impressions on adult behaviour'.

The psychological origins of both the 'confirmed criminal' and the 'chronic neuropath' were thus 'likely to be found in a misunderstood childhood'.[24]

And so, as William Moodie, psychiatrist and first Medical Director of the London Clinic put it: 'Inefficiency and unhappiness are largely promoted by the number of neurotic and psycho-neurotic adults to be found in modern life'. Such cases would be 'greatly diminished' by intervention in childhood and this was 'one of the most hopeful aspects of Child Guidance'.[25] Statements like these bear out Rose's argument that the 'child guidance clinic acted as the hub of a programmatic movement for mental hygiene' and did so through a 'powerful network linked by the activities and judgements of doctors, psychologists, probation officers and social workers'.[26]

Treatment received in such clinics would therefore benefit not only the individuals concerned but also their families and society more generally. It is worth briefly emphasizing at this juncture the wider benefits mental well-being and stability in childhood were seen to bring. In the mid-1930s it was reported, in the course of an article about the London Clinic, that: 'A well known psychologist recently said in a broadcast talk, "The problems of civilization are essentially the problems of childhood"'.[27] 'Civilization' had, of course, plenty of problems in the 1930s and one outcome of this has been noted by William Graebner. Discussing the intellectual origins of Benjamin Spock's *Common Sense Book of Baby and Child Care*, a powerful influence on post-1945 childrearing practices, Graebner notes that Spock's interest in child aggression 'was part of a widespread interest in aggression and in the relationship between individual neuroses and social disorganization' in the latter half of the 1930s.[28]

This interest was not confined to the United States. John Bowlby was, after the Second World War, to become famous for attachment theory, which stressed the importance of early infant emotional bonding with, in particular, the mother. Illustrating the tight-knit circles in which such individuals operate, Bowlby had been supervised for his doctorate by the psychologist Cyril Burt and worked under the psychiatrist Bernard Hart, another figure whose name recurs at various points in this volume.[29] In the late 1930s Bowlby did part of his psychiatric training at the London Clinic. In his co-authored book *Personal Aggressiveness and War* Bowlby clearly drew on his clinic experience, explaining how, for instance, the aggressiveness of a young male patient derived from misplaced feelings of guilt.[30] The implication was clear: reduce aggression in adulthood by addressing the issue in childhood and the collective human urge to harm others will thereby diminish. In the wake of a devastating war, and with the emergence of new international tensions in the Cold War, ensuring the emotional and psychological stability of childhood seemed, if anything, even more necessary – hence Hendrick's comment on the broader influence and significance of child guidance in the late 1940s.

Child guidance thus sought to engage not with – in the language of the time – the 'mentally deficient', nor with specifically educational problems. And although its origins lay in part with concerns about delinquency, this became less and less of an issue. Rather, child guidance addressed the problems of maladjustment in the otherwise normal child. Any child could, so the argument went, experience problems in the course of its psychological and emotional development, and failure to address these could have deleterious individual, familial and social consequences. This book's emphasis is on these normal children who attended child guidance clinics rather than those who were, for whatever reason, hospitalized or given specialized educational provision. What constituted 'normal', though, proved difficult to define with any clinical precision as did, in consequence, diagnosis and treatment.

Such difficulties notwithstanding, a staff member at the Liverpool Child Guidance Clinic, Dr Muriel Barton Hall, described her institution's client base and the symptoms they presented. 'There is', Dr Hall explained, 'in our schools a group of children whose difficulties are not so obvious because they are personality problems rather than physical problems'. The former could nonetheless be identified through 'manifestations of a behaviour disorder'. 'Such children', she continued, 'may steal, lie, wander, play truant, or defy authority, or they may show milder forms of disorder such as moodiness, solitariness, nervousness, bad habits, sleeplessness or backwardness in school subjects'.

The more extreme cases were potential criminals and might have to be dealt with by the juvenile justice system. However, the 'milder cases … although not law-breakers' were just as much in need of help 'in that so long as they are ill-adjusted they cannot contribute their full share to the life of the home, the school or the playground'.[31] It was precisely such 'milder cases' which child guidance sought to treat and in so doing to move 'behavioural disorder' out of the realm of moral failing and into that of mental health. Nonetheless, conditions such as 'solitariness' are hardly clinically precise and this was to give ammunition to those critical of the child guidance project.

If promoting mental hygiene was a major concern of child guidance, in so doing it was able to call upon the insights of the 'new psychology'. Although far from a unified or coherent movement, the 'new psychology' nonetheless had particular characteristics which were of huge significance for child guidance. As Thomson observes, 'the unconscious mind [was] now emerging as a crucial terrain for exploration'. Psychology had to recognize, moreover, that 'its subjects [were] changing rather than fixed, biological heritage in constant dialogue with environment'. Thus with 'the psychological subject so reconfigured, the door was open for psychology, not simply to record human nature, but to turn to the study of how to change it'.[32] British child guidance, like its American counterpart, was initially dominated by psychiatrists and it was this group in particular which sought to stress the necessity of understanding and employing modern psychological medicine. So, for instance, children's visible 'maladjustments' were only symptoms of deeper, underlying problems. The role of 'environment', meanwhile, was to take a pre-eminent place in child guidance diagnosis and treatment.

Here we might also note the importance of the American psychiatrist Adolf Meyer. Meyer promoted a holistic psychiatric approach which saw mental illness as caused by maladjustment between individuals and their environment. His work heavily influenced American child guidance.[33] Meyer's holistic approach was part of a much broader and influential field of medical thought. As Rosenberg observes, psychiatric holism emphasized mind–body relationships and thus the 'interactions between the internal and external environments, between the family's microenvironment and society's macroenvironment as well as between the physical and the psychological'.[34] Given that American practice and philosophy were to be at least partially 'exported' to Britain, this extends the range of Meyer's influence as well as locating it in a wider medical and intellectual culture.

Meyer is also recognized as the single most important influence on British psychiatry in the first half of the twentieth century.[35] So, for example, what was to become a standard text for British psychiatrists was dedicated to him. Equally importantly in the present context its authors, R. D. Gillespie and D. K. Henderson, were supporters of child guidance.[36] Meyer's impact is personified in Douglas MacCalman. MacCalman, supported by the Commonwealth Fund, travelled to the US to study under Meyer and one of his followers, McFie Campbell. It was on his return that he took up the Notre Dame post which started his long involvement with British child guidance.

We can find the combination of mental hygiene and the new psychology implicit in the observations of British child guidance supporters. One of these who made the trip to the United States in the late 1920s to examine child guidance practices was the Senior Medical Officer at the Board of Education, Dr Ralph Crowley. Addressing an audience on the subject of his trip, Crowley remarked that it was 'strange how vital problems, vital in the interests of the individual or the community or both, lie openly around us and yet, over a long period of years, remain unobserved and unrecognized'. Then all of a sudden, he continued, 'we are seized of them ... [and] recognize them as urgent'. Problems of emotion and behaviour among children were clearly a case in point.[37]

Child guidance's principal agency was to be the clinic where the child patient would encounter the psychiatrist, the psychologist and the PSW. The first was responsible for physical and mental examination, the second for the administration of psychological tests and the third for observing the child and its family at the clinic and at home. These three professions would thus employ their scientific expertise to ensure that the child patient be cured of the causes of his maladjustment. Parental, and especially maternal, instinct was no longer enough to ensure healthy emotional and psychological development. Expert help was needed, and given that the origins of the child's problem almost certainly derived from a malfunctioning familial environment, parents of themselves were part of the problem.[38]

The notion of 'environment' is therefore a recurring theme in this volume and for most child guidance practitioners meant not the socio-economic conditions in which the child found itself but, rather, the emotional landscape of his or her family circumstances. In child guidance practice and organization, meanwhile, much was made of the notion of 'teamwork'. Although this was in practice highly problematic in the American/medical version of child guidance which bodies such as the Commonwealth Fund and the CGC sought to promote, it was the psychiatrist who nonetheless took the lead. As Dr Barton Hall forcefully put it, it had to be accepted that 'the only safe approach to psychological diagnosis and treatment is through the science of medicine'.[39]

Promoting Child Guidance

But it was not only by way of the clinic that the child guidance message was to be spread. The CGC, for instance, put on courses for workers in children's homes with the aim of giving 'practical help in the application of modern psychological knowledge' to problems they might encounter.[40] Wider audiences were reached by, for example, the BBC radio talk given by Moodie in 1939 in a series entitled 'How They Do It Abroad'. Moodie's topic was child guidance in the United States and he both paid tribute to the role of the Commonwealth Fund in extending this work to Britain while also taking the opportunity to discuss the activities in which he and his British colleagues were engaged.[41]

All this certainly seems to have had an impact and not only in terms of the increasing number of 'patients' attending an increasing number of clinics. The 1936 conference of the National Council of Women of Great Britain urged 'the provision of Child Guidance Clinics by Education Authorities as a necessary supplement to their existing Health and Education Services'.[42] The London Teachers' Association, meanwhile, passed a resolution in 1938 expressing its appreciation of the work of London's child guidance clinics. The Association would thus 'welcome the incorporation of child guidance as a permanent feature of our educational system'.[43]

Child guidance was thus expanding institutionally and in terms of outreach by the late 1930s. The Second World War and its immediate aftermath saw its profile raised further. This was in part due to the impact of the evacuation of schoolchildren from vulnerable urban areas to the countryside and to the surveys carried out into the evacuation experience. The surveys for Scotland, for instance, noted the problems caused by some evacuated children and that, after investigation by staff from Glasgow's local authority child guidance clinics, a residential clinic had been set up. Files on those admitted, in true child guidance style, contained data on mental abilities, medical and psychiatric examinations, personal history and parental and domestic circumstances.[44]

As in the interwar era, the call for greater provision was also taken up by lay bodies and individuals. The Scottish Women's Group on Public Welfare, in an influential 1944 report, claimed that the very presence of 'problem' children among the evacuees 'indicated clearly the need for the development of the Child Guidance movement, as yet, so far as Scotland is concerned, mainly in its infancy'. Among the Group's recommendations was thus:

> That the Child Guidance Movement, with its close co-operation of Education and School Medical Services should be extensively developed, as providing in many cases a solution of the problem child's difficulties within the family before any question of a Juvenile Court arises.[45]

And in the realm of politics we find Evan Durbin, co-author with Bowlby of *Personal Aggressiveness and War* and prominent Labour Party intellectual, arguing in the 1940s for the importance of childrearing and need for improved 'emotional health'.[46] It is difficult to see such remarks as unrelated to Durbin's friendship and co-authorship with Bowlby and the latter's involvement in child guidance.

Its expansion notwithstanding, child guidance was not uncritically received. One of the commonest causes of referral to child guidance clinics was enuresis, or bed-wetting. By the interwar era how best to treat this was contested between those who sought a solution in mechanical devices which conditioned behaviour and those who supported the 'psychopathological view in which bedwetting is symptomatic of a maladjusted personality'. As Chris Hurl points out, even today the former approach is still favoured by many paediatricians. The 'psychopathological' analysis, by contrast, was very much that adopted by child guidance.[47]

Psychologists, meanwhile, resented the claims of psychiatry to leadership in the field. While psychiatry usually won out in England, at least before 1939, this was not the case in Scotland, with its historically distinct education system and methods of teacher training. Here well-entrenched educationalists and educational psychologists put up stiff resistance to what they saw as the pretensions of psychiatric medicine.[48] A leading Scottish educationalist, who himself ran a clinic for children with psychological problems and who is further encountered particularly in chapters 2 and 3, dismissively suggested that child guidance psychiatrists knew little of either education or children.[49] It is also worth asking who exactly carried out the bulk of child guidance work. While psychiatrists and psychologists might dispute professional boundaries and competences, arguably it was the PSW who had most to do with the child and its family. This was potentially problematic, at least in terms of the purported claims of child guidance, given the relatively limited nature and extent of the PSW's training.

But even within psychiatry, the particular approach which child guidance adopted was not universally accepted. Melanie Klein and Anna Freud – and their respective groups of supporters – are famed for their profound disagreements. But neither fundamentally doubted that children could be psychoanalysed, something which child guidance psychiatrists, in the early days at least, were at pains to deny occurred in child guidance clinics or was part of their approach to child mental ill-health. So, for instance, the physician E. A. Hamilton-Pearson told colleagues at the Institute of Medical Psychology in 1932 that 'psycho-analysis plays no part in our work. A child's mental conflicts are immediate and on the surface, and they must be dealt with on a commonsense basis'.[50] Such an approach has to be seen as part of a wider cultural ambiguity about psychoanalysis in interwar Britain.

A further implication of both Freudian and Kleinian approaches was that much less emphasis needed to be placed on children's emotional environment and the quality of parenting to which they were exposed. In 1927 Anna Freud told an audience that it was undoubtedly the case that the origins of a child patient's neurosis were 'not only internal, but partly external as well'. But this difference from adult neurosis was based on strictly psychoanalytical principles – the child's super-ego had not yet achieved 'independence' – and such insights only increased the significance of child analysis. Significantly, Freud's talk was entitled 'The Theory of Children's Analysis'.[51] A few years later, Melanie Klein claimed that unless parental mistakes in child rearing were 'too gross', she avoided 'interfering in the way in which the child is being brought up'.[52] Such comments also flag up an important feature of child guidance practice as it developed and as already alluded to – an increasing focus on parents and the contribution of one or the other or both to the child's maladjustment.

If professional hostility was one concern then among primary care doctors the problem, at least initially, was apathy. A report from the London Clinic in the early 1930s noted that children were mostly referred by parents and schools. There were very few referrals from doctors and this was 'a matter for regret since the Clinic is essentially a medical organization and so ought to maintain close co-operation with the medical profession'. The issue was, the report continued, that there was undoubtedly a 'feeling of distrust in the minds of many doctors as to the value and methods of psychology'. This arose because it was wrongly assumed that psychological medicine neglected some of the fundamental principles of 'scientific' medicine. Moreover physicians and surgeons felt, with some justification it was conceded, that those practicing psychological medicine looked down on organic medicine and pressed instead the claims of 'mental treatment'. This too had impacted negatively on the Clinic.[53] Nor did the coming of the National Health Service (NHS) remedy this situation. The mental health services in general continued to be understaffed and under-resourced and, as Thomson remarks, the advent of socialized health care did not 'usher in a heroic new age of psychotherapy for the masses'.[54]

Further Analysing Child Guidance

By mid-century child guidance had established itself as an important part of the mental health and social welfare provision for young people and more generally as part of the welfare state. It was also, though, a field contested by different professional groups and an area of practice and research which still sought clarity of definition and proposed outcomes. These issues are further explored in the remainder of this book. Chapter 1 examines how and why child guidance arrived in Britain and in particular the role and ambitions of the Commonwealth Fund and of the individuals and institutions to which its early support was crucial. The next chapter discusses the functions and attitudes of the various professional groups involved down to the outbreak of the Second World War and the intellectual climate in which they operated. Tensions between these groups called into question the notion of hierarchical teamwork which, at least in principle, was what was sought by advocates of the American/medical model of child guidance. The intellectual climate was shaped in part by developments in not only psychological medicine, but also in other sciences and social sciences and by broader concerns about the impact of modernity. Chapter 3 looks at the spread, down to 1939, of the child guidance message first through the medium of clinics inside and outside London including to the bastion of educational psychology, Scotland. Second, we see how the message was disseminated by professional and popular publications and meetings. In chapter 4 the focus shifts to clinics, patients and their families and asks what was meant by normalcy in childhood and whether the normal child was also a 'happy' child, which conditions or behaviours were deemed to constitute maladjustment, how these were diagnosed and treated and why it was that attention was increasingly focused on the parents – and particularly the mother – as much as on the child.

We then, in chapter 5, look at the impact of the Second World War. A key factor here was the evacuation of children from threatened urban areas and the effect this had on perceptions of child mental health as well as on the children themselves. Notwithstanding the constraints imposed on the wartime provision of child guidance, this nonetheless increased. In chapter 6 we analyse the outcome of the development of child guidance over the preceding two decades through its embedding in the welfare state by way of the Education Acts. Despite the promotion of the medical model by influential groups, the nature of child guidance's incorporation into the welfare state allowed psychology to claim the territory it had long sought. Chapter 7 thus returns to the issue of professional groups and their respective roles in child guidance provision in these changing circumstances. This also allows for a further investigation of the clinic experience as well as an analysis of the Underwood Report, the evidence given to it and how its findings were received. The concluding chapter draws all these strands together under six thematic heads and assesses the success or otherwise of child guidance in its formative first three decades by, for example, engaging with the critical contemporary assessment by the prominent social scientist Barbara Wootton. An attempt is also made to judge to what degree child guidance actually helped children and their parents or whether it was, for instance, simply a further contribution to familial, and especially maternal, anxiety. To what degree, then, did child guidance help children and their parents navigate, in the words of one psychiatrist, 'The Dangerous Age of Childhood'?[55] Or to put it another way, why were some children, in a phrase encountered earlier in this chapter, an enigma to their parents?

This sense of the enigmatic child, the anxieties engendered by parenthood and the threats to both parent and child are captured in Mervyn Jones's novel of working-class London life in the first half of the twentieth century, *Holding On*. In the years just before the Second World War the heroine, Ann, is particularly concerned about one of her sons, Harry. Harry was 'a quiet child, rather shy, rather withdrawn' and mildly troublesome at school. His mother felt that 'it was difficult to understand what went on in Harry's mind – or in Harry's feelings, the well-defended heart of him'. Despite the assertions to the contrary of her husband and a friend, Ann felt that it was impossible 'to worry too much' about her children's development. Consequently she 'read the advice columns in the women's weeklies, and worked her way through books by psychologists from the public library'. These made her realize the 'harm that could be done by a small mishap' such as speaking harshly to your child, something which resulted in Harry withdrawing into 'unexplained misery'. For Ann, then, 'a happy child was a gift of luck, flourishing in the face of reason and probability like a tree on a waste ground'.[56]

Although, of course, a piece of fiction, this passage nonetheless captures many of the issues which we shall encounter in subsequent chapters: the 'problem' of shyness and similar sorts of behaviour, the lack of understanding on the parent's part of the working of the child's mind, Ann's attempt to redress this through advice columns and reading psychology books, the unintended consequences, notably unhappiness, of parental actions and the general sense of inadequacy and unease, the latter in particular being part of the broader cultural and intellectual climate of the period dealt with in this volume.

1 CHILD GUIDANCE COMES TO BRITAIN

Introduction

For exponents of child guidance, children's behavioural problems were to be dealt with not on the basis of moral judgement but rather through the application of science, and in particular medical science. Earlier work on delinquency and developments in the psychology of individual difference, meanwhile, had drawn attention to the behaviour of the whole child population. To address the perceived problems required the employment of professional expertise. As a Child Guidance Council publication of the late 1920s put it, a child guidance clinic was 'not primarily a "place", though, of course, it must have a location; it is primarily a <u>specially trained staff</u>' (emphasis in original). The same pamphlet also noted that at present to 'see these clinics in full working order, we must turn to America, the home of the Child Guidance Clinic' and that it was the Commonwealth Fund which was crucial in advancing child guidance, both in the US and in Britain.[1] Similarly admiring of the American example was an article in the journal of the Froebel Society, *Child Life*, which remarked that the possibility of the 'readjustment' of the 'problem child' had been 'amply proved' by American clinics. Hence 'a study of their methods', which had passed beyond 'the first experimental stage', should 'help [child guidance practitioners] to forward such work in England'.[2]

We therefore examine the emergence of child guidance in America after the First World War and its spread thereafter. The role of the Commonwealth Fund is analysed, including its part in enabling British observers to visit America to witness child guidance in action. The Fund was also instrumental in the setting up of three other key elements in the early history of British child guidance: the CGC, the London Clinic and the Diploma in Mental Health course at the London School of Economics (LSE).

The Origins of Child Guidance

Child guidance emerged in the United States in the immediate aftermath of the First World War. It did not arrive, however, from nowhere.[3] Virtually all accounts of the establishment of child guidance, American and British, note the significance of the physician William Healy who was co-founder, in 1909, of the Chicago-based Juvenile Psychopathic Institute. The Institute's aim was to understand delinquency's psychological origins through the study of individual young offenders. Healy and his colleagues in Progressive Era campaigns for child welfare reform were, albeit to differing degrees, alert to the significance of the child's familial environment. As Jones remarks, this sort of approach exemplified the 'unique Progressive blend of scientific investigation that often motivated reformers to turn to the medical sciences for help with social problems'.[4]

Among the intellectual influences on Healy were the pioneering child psychologist G. Stanley Hall and the psychiatrist Adolf Meyer. The latter argued against mind–body dualism and instead for 'psychobiology', wherein the whole person was diagnosed and treated. For Meyer mental illness was caused by 'a lack of fit, or maladjustment, between the individual and the environment'.[5] There was therefore, and very much in line with trends in psychiatry which sought to stress its broader social relevance and intervention, a need to move beyond the asylum. Meyer was instrumental in founding, in the US, the National Committee for Mental Hygiene. This aspired to promote mental health and in so doing emphasized the centrality of childhood and, ultimately, of child guidance. As Meyer put it in a speech to American social workers in 1925, the National Committee 'has been enabled to establish its child guidance clinics, nominally for the prevention of delinquency, but really a step toward reaching the broader needs of health, happiness, efficiency, and social adaptation'.[6]

Meyer's comments reveal, wittingly and otherwise, much about the aspirations of mental hygiene and child guidance. Both clearly had social as well as medical ambitions with a view to, in the case of child guidance, ensuring the successful integration of the child with its wider environment. Adaptation was to be achieved by positive intervention to counter maladjustment and thereby to promote individual, familial and social harmony. Meyer's audience was also significant. He had used social workers in his own clinics – part of his strategy of seeing the 'whole' person – prior to the First World War, as had other institutions. But one particularly important development was the setting up of a course in psychiatric social work at Smith College, Massachusetts, in 1918. Further expansion came with the foundation of the Institute for Child Guidance in New York which provided specialized facilities for Smith College students.[7] This new profession was to be central to the development of child guidance with the first cohort of British psychiatric social workers coming to the US for training. Thus

British child guidance sought to adopt American practices, ideas and ambitions albeit it with important national variations.

But Meyer's remarks omit one further crucial actor in American child guidance's history. In 1921 a conference in New Jersey brought together a group of experts in delinquency. This meeting was supported by the Commonwealth Fund and the outcome was that the Fund agreed to support the setting up of training – most notably at the Institute for Child Guidance – and clinic facilities for what was known, from 1922, as 'child guidance'. As Jones observes, this was an important point in the shift from a concern primarily with delinquents to a focus on difficult non-delinquents while also illustrating child guidance's 'close adherence to the individual, psychological paradigm of troublesome behaviour'.[8]

At first glance all this would seem to be of concern principally to historians of American childhood. However this would be to neglect the international exchange of ideas in social reform characteristic of the first few decades of the twentieth century. Daniel Rodgers argues that in historical writing the 'narrative field too often shrinks back on the nation; the boundaries of the nation-state become an analytical cage'. One area where such an approach is particularly inappropriate, he continues, is in American 'social politics' in the Progressive and New Deal eras when, 'as every contemporary who followed these issues knew', the reconstruction of social politics 'was of a part with movements of politics and ideas throughout the North Atlantic'. In consequence such social politics had their origins 'not in its nation-state containers, not in a hypothesized "Europe" nor an equally imagined "America", but in the world between them'.[9] Rodgers's case is somewhat overstated – national differences were important in child welfare policies as in other areas of social politics – but he has a point about international awareness of developments in particular fields and the willingness to adopt and adapt ideas from abroad.

So, for instance, it has been shown that the first Dutch child guidance clinic was 'modelled after the American example', that the woman jurist who set up this institution was to go on to revive the Dutch National Association for Mental Health and that she had drawn inspiration from a trip to the US in the early 1920s when she had visited, among other institutions, the New York Child Guidance Clinic.[10] Ultimately, and as elsewhere, this was to shift the emphasis in Dutch child welfare from the primarily moral to the primarily medical.[11] In Norway, meanwhile, child guidance slowly emerged in the interwar era, influenced by American and British precedents.[12]

As the last point suggests, Europeans sought to learn from each other as well as from the United States. Immediately prior to becoming medical director of the Birmingham Child Guidance Clinic in 1933, C. L. C. Burns toured Europe to observe child guidance in no less than seven nations. Burns noted both common patterns and national differences, the latter attributable to, inter alia, 'racial' distinctions and, more importantly, the degree of emphasis placed on the medical versus the psychological approach.[13] Like mental hygiene, and unsurprisingly given the relationship between the two, the development of child guidance was thus an international phenomenon after 1918 and one in which different nations sought to learn from each other. This was to operate partly through the movement of psychiatrists, psychologists and PSWs across national boundaries to study other countries' principles and practice.

To return to American influences we might note the remarks of the Director of the East London Child Guidance Clinic who commended the 'investigations of Healey [*sic*] in Chicago' for establishing 'the relationship between social milieu and mental maladjustment'.[14] The psychologist G. Stanley Hall, meanwhile, was an important intellectual influence on the British Child Study movement from the 1890s. Although the latter petered out in the early twentieth century it helped to create, as Hendrick puts it, a situation wherein 'medical psychologists and doctors were defining children in an apparently "scientific" manner, thereby making it difficult for lay persons to dispute their findings'.[15]

The Commonwealth Fund of New York

And, of course, we have the role and aspirations of the Commonwealth Fund, set up in 1918 with the general aim of doing, in the words of its founders, 'something for the welfare of mankind'.[16] Its president during the interwar era was Edward Harkness, an Anglophile known for his interest in education, scientific medicine and child welfare.[17] Harkness's chief administrator was Barry Smith, a trained social worker and, like Harkness, a Yale graduate.[18] The Fund's initial bequest was $10 million and from the early 1930s it devoted the bulk of its activities to medicine, broadly defined, although even before then it had had a strong bias in this direction.[19]

The Fund's approach was part of a more general trend in American philanthropy. Emily Rosenberg comments that after 1918 the religious impulse which had originally shaped American philanthropy gave way to a 'secularized emphasis on uplift and science and technology'. This was not, moreover, simply confined to foundation activities in the US but was equally central to their 'Missions to the world'.[20] David Hammack argues that the Commonwealth Fund and the other major foundations 'committed themselves in the early 1920s to scientific and medical research and to efforts to place the health-care, education, and social-service professions on a scientific non-sectarian basis'.[21] And, in a contemporary comment, Elizabeth Macadam found the Fund's support of British child guidance an instance of the 'new philanthropy' she saw emerging in the interwar era.[22] Before examining the key role undoubtedly played by the Commonwealth Fund, though, it is necessary to make two qualifications.

First, we have already noted that child guidance was a contested field and not least in the respective aspirations of psychiatry and psychology. So in Scotland a psychologist and an educationalist were, from the mid-1920s, operating clinics for children with behavioural problems. Although these were not at the time designated as dealing with 'child guidance' the two individuals involved, James Drever and William Boyd, were later to claim theirs were among the first British child guidance clinics. Drever and Boyd feature prominently in our account of the resistance of psychology to psychiatry's claims over child guidance. In this they followed the example and inspiration of their intellectual mentor, Cyril Burt. Burt had worked extensively on delinquency and his status was recognized by his appointment in 1913 to the London County Council (LCC). He was to be a presence, if often a strangely muted one, in British child guidance history. The central point remains, though, that psychologists took an early interest in child guidance. The Committee for Research in Education of the British Psychological Society (BPS) noted in 1929 the need for research in areas such as the 'nature, frequency, and treatment of neurotic children' while later the same year the psychologist Lucy Fildes, soon to be a tutor on the LSE Diploma in Mental Health course, gave a talk to the BPS's Education Committee on 'Child Guidance Clinics'.[23]

Second, there were certain psychiatric initiatives which pre-dated Commonwealth Fund involvement. The Institute for Medical Psychology – later the Tavistock Clinic – was established by the psychiatrist Hugh Crichton-Miller in 1920. As its historian notes, the Institute's emphasis in the pursuit of mental hygiene was on 'understanding the patient as the product of his own environment and of his own history'. From the beginning there was a separate clinic for children and an emphasis on the multi-disciplinary team of psychiatrist, psychologist and social worker. Indeed the first patient seen at the Tavistock was a child and this was therefore 'some years before the first "official" Child Guidance Clinic opened in London'.[24] Like all the early clinics, though, the Tavistock survived thanks to voluntary contributions. A report from 1931 noted this point and that its children's clinic medical staff received only nominal fees. Nonetheless the Tavistock was an important institution, and the report also noted the participation on its Medical Advisory Board of leading child guidance proponents such as Moodie and Henderson.[25]

In 1925, meanwhile, the Jewish Health Organization set up the East London Child Guidance Clinic under the supervision of the ubiquitous Emanuel Miller. Although this clinic was to receive certain forms of support from the Commonwealth Fund via the CGC, essentially it too was an independent body. As such it was the forerunner of those clinics which, during the interwar period, gained varying degrees of indirect subsidy from the Commonwealth Fund but also had to seek financial and other forms of support from other sources. The establish-

ment of the East London Clinic was also important in that Miller was to be a
consistent advocate of the medical approach to child guidance and because his
co-workers included Sybil Clement Brown, soon to be a leading figure in British
psychiatric social work and a key contributor to debates about the nature and
direction of child guidance.[26]

To return to the Commonwealth Fund, the key ways in which it promoted
British child guidance were through the CGC and the London Clinic, observational and training trips to the USA and the Diploma in Mental Health at
the LSE. How did this situation come about and what did the Fund expect in
return? In 1925 the English magistrate Anne St Loe Strachey observed the work
of the Philadelphia Child Guidance Clinic during a trip to the US. This was
one of the institutions supported by the Commonwealth Fund and particularly
prominent in the promotion of the child guidance message.[27] On her return she
contacted the Fund and consequently again visited the US in 1926 to inspect
various child guidance institutions and to meet with Barry Smith and his assistant Mildred Scoville, another trained social worker. St Loe Strachey had been
convinced of the need to extend child guidance to Britain arguing that although
the latter had psychiatric clinics, none fully corresponded to those available in
the US.[28] As a result, Smith told Edward Harkness, he was sending Scoville to
Britain to assess the situation.[29] For the whole of its relationship with British
child guidance Scoville was to be the Fund's key intermediary.

Prior to her departure, and highlighting child guidance's international dimensions, Scoville was approached by the American professional body for PSWs
asking whether in Scoville's view it could make 'new contacts of value in England'.
The correspondent further noted a parallel move in Germany to establish psychiatric social work.[30] Scoville was also in correspondence with Evelyn Fox, another
leading proponent of British child guidance as well as a prominent figure in the
Central Association for Mental Welfare and, shortly thereafter, a member of the
Wood Committee on Mental Deficiency. Fox had clearly compiled a demanding
itinerary for Scoville's visit. But the latter seemed to accept this, remarking that she
wished to learn about work in psychiatry, psychology and mental hygiene alongside associated activities dealing with, especially, children. Scoville also wished to
be apprised of training facilities for social workers.[31] Reporting to Smith on her
trip, Scoville claimed that there was 'no doubt' that in general the US was ahead
in dealing with 'problem children' and not least in social work training. 'It seems
to me', she concluded, 'that this is the psychological time to lay the foundations
for the development of child guidance work in England; and the most important need is undoubtedly the development of specialized training for this field'.[32]
Scoville further suggested to Smith that a British delegation should visit the US
in advance of any child guidance programme being started.[33]

The Founding of the Child Guidance Council

At this stage British proponents of child guidance appear to have been organized through the English Child Guidance Committee and an informal meeting seems to have taken place involving this body, the National Council for Mental Hygiene, the Central Association for Mental Welfare, the Magistrates' Association and the Howard League for Penal Reform.[34] As a document apparently emanating from the Committee noted, the initiative had been taken by St Loe Strachey. In turn, this led to 'a small group of people in this country' devising a scheme 'which could be set on foot if the Commonwealth Fund were prepared to finance the project'.[35] In response the Fund agreed that it might be prepared to support a plan for

> the improvement of facilities for the handling of problem children through the development of a training center in which [trained] social workers, psychiatrists and psychologists ... can receive practical training and experience in clinical work with children from the mental hygiene point of view.

Various conditions were attached including financial viability, robust organizational structures, appropriate academic links and the 'staffing of the clinic wholly or chiefly by English personnel' and it was again urged that key British child guidance advocates visit the US for at least, in each individual's case, three months.[36] Commenting on this interventionist revision of the British proposals, Smith told Harkness that '[w]e are convinced that the proposition is a sound one and that the opportunity for doing a real service is quite unusual'. Presciently anticipating trouble with his future British collaborators, Smith also remarked that while the scheme, particularly if Scoville could work closely with the British, 'should unquestionably be successful' nonetheless '[w]e are also convinced it will not be an easy thing to work out'.[37]

Fund engagement with British child guidance now began to gain momentum. Smith told Harkness in early 1927 that the committee had changed its name to the Child Guidance Council and that the latter had agreed to his proposals. This apparent good news was again tempered by problems on the British side, almost exclusively over finance. The Fund, like all American philanthropies, saw financial intervention as being of a clearly limited duration with local sources ultimately taking over. As Smith remarked there were grounds to 'question ... the ability of the English group to finance the clinic on a permanent basis after the demonstration period'. 'I am not clear', he continued, 'as to whether this phase of the subject has been evaded or whether they simply feel that it is not possible to make such decisions at the present time'.[38]

Reservations notwithstanding, this was an important moment. The CGC, the principle mechanism through which Commonwealth Fund monies were to be disbursed and the body which saw itself as having the key strategic role in promoting a particular version of child guidance, had been established. Collectively and individually, the Council vigorously promoted its ideas. So, for instance, Evelyn Fox wrote to Sir George Newman, Chief Medical Officer (CMO) at the Board of Education, outlining Fund and CGC plans for a clinic. But if such institutions were to be a 'permanent part of child care in this country', she continued, then 'they must eventually be under the aegis of the Education Authorities'. Fox also raised the question of whether clinic attendance would count towards school attendance, for her a 'vital issue' in advancing child guidance.[39] These were on the face of it simply administrative matters, but they were to have a profound effect on the way in which British child guidance developed.

By the late 1920s the Council boasted an impressive membership including the psychiatrists Hugh Crichton-Miller and R. G. Gordon, the social scientists C. M. Lloyd and A. M. Carr-Saunders and the psychologists C. E. Spearman and Cyril Burt. Professional and other bodies represented included the British Medical Association (BMA), the Social Hygiene Council, the National Council for Mental Hygiene, the LCC and the Royal Medico-Psychological Society. Three government departments were also represented – the Home Office, the Board of Education and the Board of Control.[40] The committee which carried out negotiations with the Commonwealth Fund was especially high-powered and included Burt, Crichton-Miller, Professor Godfrey Thomson of the Education Department at Edinburgh University and H. W. Shawcross, Secretary of the Howard League and future Cabinet Minister.[41]

Another influential Council member was Priscilla Norman, later wife of the governor of the Bank of England and author of a memoir which gives intriguing insights into the Council's workings. Norman felt that her own unhappy childhood had led her to child guidance work when she began to realize, in adulthood, that 'many other children had shared my plight, and that there was a scientific explanation which the experts in this child guidance business were beginning to unravel'. Norman's use of the words 'scientific' and 'experts' here is revealing, suggesting that as a lay person she had bought into these aspects of child guidance. Among her fellow lay Council members was Ramsay MacDonald's daughter, Ishbel, who when her father became prime minister 'was always ready to help by lending No. 10 for meetings or fund raising concerns'.[42]

The Council's role and status was publicly recognized by the Commonwealth Fund. The 1928 Report of the General Director (i.e. Smith), for instance, remarked that its members included 'important lay members of high social standing and wide influence'.[43] This was not simply a matter of snobbery. The need for individuals of high political and social status – Norman and MacDonald being obvious examples – was deemed essential for efficient fund-raising. The 1929 annual report similarly observed that the Council had become a 'strong, active, and responsible organization, highly representative of all groups concerned with the mental and physical health and welfare of children'.[44] More than this, though, the Council's creation had stimulated British child guidance in four further ways.

The first and most obvious of these was financial. The Council's consolidation and its apparent willingness to be at least to some extent directed by the Fund in turn led the latter to commit itself to the development of child guidance in Britain. As the 1929 annual report further noted, the Council had been 'supported thus far entirely by the Commonwealth Fund'.[45] The Fund now saw child guidance as the central constituent of its English [*sic*] Mental Hygiene Program and was to do so, albeit with increasing reluctance, down to 1945. To give some scale of the commitment, the 1929 General Director's Report noted that some $68,500 had been appropriated to this end.[46] Funding peaked in 1933/4 at just over $86,500, staying around (on average) $60,000 per annum for the rest of the 1930s before declining during the 1940s.[47] Monies available to the CGC were to be used in various ways including scholarships and fellowships for psychiatrists, psychologists and PSWs and support to clinics outside London. So, for example, the accounts for 1933 record a grant to the Liverpool clinic of £50 and just under £1,000 devoted to fellowships.[48] Equally important, though, was the 'loan' system for PSWs discussed further in chapter 3.

Observing American Child Guidance

The second way in which the Fund helped to establish British child guidance was through the visit to the US, in 1927, of eight leading individuals drawn from a range of professions and interests. These included the prominent psychiatrist Bernard Hart, the medical doctors Letitia Fairfield and Ralph Crowley, the renowned psychologist Charles Spearman and the social worker Miss St Clair Townsend. Their various comments on their experiences are illuminating and suggest how the American model of child guidance, assiduously promoted by the Commonwealth Fund, was articulated by these visitors to a wider British audience.

Collectively, the visitors submitted a report to the CGC. This argued for the necessity of linking potential clinics with Local Education Authorities (LEAs), close relationships, where possible, with local hospitals and the need for specialist training for all staff. The document crucially concurred with the dominant American view that 'the Head of the Clinic should be a psychiatrist' while stressing 'the necessity for and adequate staff of specially trained social workers, as they are an indispensable part of the Clinic'.[49] Individuals also submitted reports on their particular specialisms. St Clair Townsend remarked that the 'rapid growth and development' of American psychiatric social work in the last decade 'is one of the most striking facts in the history of Mental Hygiene work'. Anticipating the need to spread the child guidance message in Britain, she further commented that one of the 'fundamental principles' she had discerned in America was that 'the Clinic should serve as a centre for disseminating knowledge in the treatment of difficult children by training workers, giving public lectures, and undertaking cooperative work with other agencies'.[50]

Dr Fairfield, meanwhile, reported back to her LCC employers. She described the workings of the Cleveland clinic and the role of the PSW. The latter could, for instance, take a case further than the psychiatrist would be able to directly through measures such as 'the breaking down of a foolish mother's favouritism for a petted child'. The claim that too much emotional attention was as bad as too little was a recurrent theme in child guidance history. The value of the social worker's report, Fairfield observed, 'lies not only in the thoroughness of American case histories but in the "psychiatric outlook" of the compiler'. In other words, the social worker was to be specially trained. This was part of Fairfield's more general view of the need to professionalize social work and that opposition to this as, for example, from the chairman of the Board of Control was discriminatory. Lest any of this alarm her readers Fairfield continued that:

> In view of the very lively dread of psycho-analysis in certain quarters, it may be said here that I did not find anything approaching analysis being carried on at any clinic. Most of the staff were not Freudians, but behaviourists, and even in the few cases where the psychiatrists belonged to the analytic school they did not think the procedure suitable for clinic conditions.

She also noted, and again this was to be a characteristic of British child guidance, that the 'general tendency' was to not directly interfere with the child's mental process but rather to seek to alter them through 'the adults who are in a natural relation of authority to him ... and through other environmental factors'.[51]

The psychologist Spearman – who had visited a wide range of clinics, including those in New York and Philadelphia – noted without direct comment that in the US it was the norm for the psychiatrist to be in charge of the clinic and that consequently 'the duties of the psychologist are mainly of a psychometrical kind'. Nonetheless, and somewhat contradicting himself, he remarked that in an 'unexpectedly large' number of cases treatment consisted of adjustment of the child's school environment and here the brunt of the work was undertaken by the psychologist. Most frequently of all, though, the 'recommended treatment concerns mostly the child's home life and environment; here, the supervision is undertaken by the social worker'. Concluding, and in an observation which was to hold increasingly true of British child guidance, Spearman remarked that: 'Much more often than not, a case which has begun by seeking to modify the behaviour of a child has developed into trying primarily to modify the behaviour of his parents'.[52]

Perhaps the most comprehensive account of an investigative trip came from Ralph Crowley in his speech to the British Association for the Advancement of Science in late 1928. Crowley reviewed previous educational legislation and how a recent focus on delinquent children had 'opened our eyes to the importance of behaviour in children generally'. In turn this had led to a concern for maladjusted children who could be 'found among children of every degree of intellectual capacity'. This was, in other words, a group markedly different from both the delinquent and the 'retarded'. Crowley then turned to his American experience. He paid tribute to the pioneering work of Healy, Meyer, the National Committee for Mental Hygiene and the Commonwealth Fund before focusing on child guidance organization and philosophy. Crowley acknowledged American child guidance's diversity but also found strong underlying similarities between clinics and various forms of practice and approach. So, for instance, clinics were generally staffed by psychiatrists, psychologists and psychiatric social workers and teamwork was seen as essential. Similarly, there were consistent patterns in the type of child referred. As to the philosophy behind child guidance, Crowley pressed home the idea that it had come into being because 'workers in the field of mental hygiene' had come to realize that behavioural problems in youth and adulthood had not arisen 'as bolts from the blue'. Rather, such problems often had their roots in earlier life. Crowley was thus anxious to stress child guidance's research dimension while noting that treatment was a process 'in conception scientific, in form an art, and one involving much patience and understanding on the part of those concerned'.[53]

Turning to the situation at home Crowley acknowledged that there was as yet no real equivalent of American child guidance. Nonetheless there were solid foundations on which British supporters could build – the work of the Tavistock Clinic and of the Jewish Clinic as well as Burt's leadership of the LCC psychological services. He also raised a problematic issue which was to persist throughout the period under consideration and which we saw flagged up by Fox. There was no doubt, he suggested, that child guidance was a branch of medicine dealing with mental health. On the other hand, 'the channels of healing' were primarily to be found through the 'manifold services of education'. Crowley therefore predicted that Britain would, at least organizationally, differ from the US by having 'a more direct and organic connection with the educational and with the school medical and infant welfare systems of the area' – that is, with local authorities. But however it was organized, what was central was that child guidance, with input from the three professions involved, was necessary 'not only from the point of view of efficient education in the narrower sense, but from that of general healthy development upon which social welfare ultimately depends'. Finally, Crowley noted the founding of the CGC and the planned London Clinic. The latter had had three years' financial support promised by the Commonwealth Fund, a body to which, Crowley remarked, 'the child guidance and the whole mental hygiene movement owe so much'.[54]

The London Clinic

The next key development in British child guidance's early history was the setting up of the London Clinic. The London County Council had shown a consistent interest in the development of child guidance and had been approached in June 1927 by the CGC for support in setting up a clinic. A decision on this had been deferred until Fairfield's return from America. In May 1928 an LCC subcommittee consequently considered her report. It was decided, in the light of the latter, to approve the original proposal for an experimental period, to gain LCC representation on the CGC and to have the clinic recognized for educational purposes. It was also agreed that there should be no charge for children referred.[55] Priscilla Norman throws further light on these events. Her interest in child guidance had started when she was a member of the LCC and, in 1927, first heard of developments in America. She had put a paper to the Council on the subject, which was opposed by the ruling party, Municipal Reform, to which Norman herself belonged, but was supported by the Labour Party and progressive doctors and educationalists in Council employment. Successful pressure from those in favour of child guidance had helped enable the participation of LCC employees in the visit to the United States.[56]

Two further significant developments concerning the LCC took place in 1928. First, the Board of Education agreed that the London Clinic be recognized for educational purposes, an issue earlier raised by Fox and Crowley. This apparently minor technical matter was important for school attendance purposes and thereby finance and, more generally, because it signalled the Board's first direct involvement in child guidance.[57] So the Board's CMO welcomed the proposed setting up of the clinic, its cooperation with the LCC and the Commonwealth Fund's financial support of both the clinic and the American visit by Crowley, a Board employee.[58] The Board's engagement at this early stage anticipated its further role in the mid-1930s and child guidance's embedding in the welfare state as a primarily educational, rather than medical, service. The second development was the LCC's agreement that three of its non-medical staff be given a year's leave of absence, financially underwritten by the Commonwealth Fund, to study psychiatric social work in New York. Among these was Noel Hunnybun, who was to go on to be a prominent PSW, secretary of the CGC, tutor on the LSE Diploma in Mental Health course, officer of the Association of Psychiatric Social Workers and leading figure in British child guidance generally.[59]

It is worth pausing our discussion of the London Clinic's development to examine two of these aspects of Hunnybun's career, as they throw considerable light on the direction in which the more psychiatrically inclined proponents of British child guidance wanted the field to move. While training in the US, Hunnybun received glowing reports from her tutors. At the Institute for Child

Guidance in New York she was seen as 'an efficient, sensitive, fine person, with a capacity for leadership'. Hunnybun had had a case load which involved 'intensive analytical work'. She had, moreover,

> completed new histories, analyzed social, psychologic [*sic*] and psychiatric material, participated in conferences and carried through treatment. Her cases have included children from six and one-half years to eighteen years, who have shown emotional problems of adolescence, response to parental difficulties, unsatisfactory relationships between parent and child, and school unadjustment [*sic*].[60]

By the time of Hunnybun's return it is clear that the Commonwealth Fund was becoming increasingly disenchanted with Evelyn Fox's attitude and behavior, to the extent that one official visitor to England had threatened to withdraw Fund support for British child guidance. The same visitor then had a discussion with Hunnybun who complained of Fox's 'domineering attitude', that all those who had returned from training in the United States had been 'consistently kept in the dark' and that 'whenever any of them said anything or expressed an opinion Miss Fox promptly overruled them on the ground that they had become Americanized and that American methods were no good in England'. Hunnybun consequently wanted Fox 'eliminated from the picture'.[61] Although Fox was far from eliminated she did duly resign as Secretary of the CGC, to the palpable relief of Fund officials, with Hunnybun succeeding. The immediate grounds for her resignation, although clearly it had been a long time coming, were her belief that social workers should be predominantly volunteers and that research and practice in mental deficiency should be part of child guidance.[62]

What we get a flavour of in the first of these episodes is the nature of training received in America and its heavily psychiatric orientation. In fact, this was a source of considerable discomfort for some visitors. Evelyn Lawrence was in the same cohort as Hunnybun. The report on her suggested that while in one case she had utilized 'ego–libido' theory, in another she had been disconcerted when the child's parents seemed 'more concerned with discussing their own problems than in telling about [the] patient'. Lawrence admitted 'some sensitivity about intimate information on marital situations [and] was at first rather overwhelmed by the frankness of these parents. She has discussed her own problems and is handling same. It is too early to gauge results'.[63] It is nonetheless clear from the second episode that Hunnybun and other proponents of the medical model sought to import psychiatrically informed social work to Britain and that this was resisted by more traditional and voluntarist social reformers such as Fox. The latter was also out of step with Fund aspirations and taken together the two suggest the desire on the part of individuals such as Hunnybun to professionalize and medicalize British child guidance and move it away from what had been up to that point a rather amateurish and ad hoc approach. More generally it is also important to stress the central role of psychiatric social work in professionalizing social work as a whole, not least through what was a purportedly more rigorous form of training.

But to return to the London Clinic, this opened in July 1929.[64] As the *British Medical Journal* (*BMJ*) reported the clinic, situated in Islington, would soon be receiving patients for treatment. It was housed 'in an attractive building having a pleasant garden, and is near the chief university and medical schools'. The latter point alludes to the training function which the clinic was also to have. It was here, in other words, that many among the early generations of child guidance professionals were to receive their induction into the field's techniques and philosophy. The journal also noted, as was by now routine, the Commonwealth Fund's generosity, that the LCC was cooperating with the clinic which also had Board of Education approval and that it was to be staffed by a team of psychiatrists, psychologists and psychiatric social workers.[65]

Among this team were Hunnybun and Moodie. Hunnybun had been seconded from the LCC at the CGC's request.[66] Moodie, formerly of the Maudsley Hospital, was appointed director. He was later described by Bowlby as 'an avuncular figure who had been appointed as a safe man whose common-sense approach would be acceptable in influential quarters'.[67] Moodie actively sought a high profile for the clinic throughout his tenure as director. Around the time of the clinic's opening a session was held on child guidance at the Congress of the Royal Sanitary Institute, suggesting both more widespread professional interest in the topic and the evangelizing of its supporters. Those who spoke were Moodie, Crowley, Fox and the Birmingham School Medical Officer, Dr G. A. Auden.[68] The last speaker (also the father of the poet W. H. Auden) is noteworthy in that Birmingham was going to be in the vanguard of the spread of child guidance outside London, and because he was to continue to contribute to analyses of child maladjustment.

Also in mid-1929, Moodie published an important article in a non-clinical journal which laid out the new institution's aims and working practices. The roles of the three professions involved are discussed more fully in the next chapter, but Moodie's piece highlights early perceptions of each of these professions from the perspective of a leading child guidance psychiatrist. It is thus worth considering at this point. Emphasizing the centrality of his own profession and the clinic's adherence thereby to the American model promoted by the Commonwealth Fund, Moodie described the psychiatrist as the 'chief' of the clinic team who was in full charge of individual cases and with team members working under his direction. As such he would, for example, chair case conferences, at the end of which he had the 'duty of summing up and deciding future policy' in respect of individual patients. Moodie was also at pains to stress the shift which had taken place in psychiatry. Previously a psychiatrist had been a physician who was 'merely ... experienced in the care of the insane, and the diagnosis of their ailments'. Now, though, psychiatry embraced a much wider field 'including the maintenance of mental health'. It was thus recognized that while much could be learned from the study of mental disease there was 'infinitely more profit in the observation of those very minor variations from normal which occur in all of us from time to time'.[69]

This last point was crucial. A key contention of child guidance was that any child, however apparently normal, could at some point become maladjusted. Concern with what constituted 'normal' became a central, and ultimately unresolved, component of British child guidance. But, as Moodie noted, these were early days. The very expression 'child guidance' was, he conceded, problematic in that it both failed to convey adequately 'the range of its subject' while giving rise to 'misconceptions as to its nature and scope'. Moodie has here unwittingly posed a question which was ultimately to haunt child guidance – what exactly was it, and what did it seek to do? However, at least in the late 1920s, the expression had been widely accepted as broadly meaning 'the sum total of the activities directed towards the Mental Hygiene of the young and, in particular, the name ... applied to a certain type of clinic which has been devised as a centre for these activities'.[70] So for Moodie his own profession was reinventing itself and applying itself to (admittedly somewhat amorphous) projects such as child guidance in which psychiatrists were taking a leading role.

What, though, of the other team members? Psychologists had the task of carrying out psychometric tests. However, the 'skilled psychologist' could contribute more than simply an IQ score through observing how the child patient actually went about tackling these tests. Such observations could 'give invaluable pointers in the summing up of the case'. Implicitly, then, the psychologist had some form of clinical role. But it was the PSWs' responsibilities which Moodie was at pains to stress. The utilization of these 'specially trained social workers' was, he suggested, 'probably the greatest advance which has been made in the constitution of the clinic team'. Moodie dismissed as unfounded popular fears that the social worker's home investigations were intrusive, emphasizing instead the creation of a positive relationship with the child and its family. Indeed, through such a relationship there was 'no doubt that she can render a much truer account of the home environmental factors than a psychiatrist can ever obtain from the parents over his consulting room table'. This assessment of the home environment was crucial since another underlying child guidance principle was that maladjustment generally arose from dysfunction in domestic, and particularly parent–child, relationships. A further implication of this was thus that the social worker was also a 'very valuable adjunct in treatment'. Such treatment consisted of 'modifying the environment rather than in any attempt to influence directly the child's conduct by psychotherapy' although the latter might occasionally be used for older children. It was, therefore, in dealing directly with the parents that the PSW had a particular role to play. In so modifying the environment it was of 'supreme importance to foster and not to frustrate tendencies such as self-restraint and a feeling of personal responsibility, without which no child can ever become a good citizen'.[71]

Moodie was thus arguing that a stable childhood was a necessary prerequisite of responsible adult citizenship. More than this, though, it was fundamental to child guidance that a maladjusted child would have a deleterious effect on its family and that this in turn would contribute to social instability. Child guidance was hence a form of preventive medicine with a social mission. The broader context here was interwar threats to liberal democracy from authoritarian movements and economic depression, the upheavals of the Second World War and the post-war emphasis on social reconstruction with the family as a key institution. Moodie's emphasis on certain desirable behavioural attributes – personal responsibility and self-restraint – also flags up another consistent theme, the perceived need for emotional moderation.

Moodie, unwittingly, raised further issues about child guidance which were to recur over the next three decades. In reality, for instance, how 'psychiatric' was it that the profession having most contact with the child, its family and its home environment was the PSW? As shall be argued in the next chapter, the training of this newly formed profession may indeed have been more sophisticated than that of more generalist social workers, but it was still far short of that of a medically trained psychiatrist. Moreover, given that the focus was increasingly as much on the child's family as on the child itself, is child guidance not a further example in welfare history where the initial focus on the child slips into a focus on parenting? This was certainly, by Margo Horn's account, what happened in the US. Horn also remarks that American child guidance can be seen as being driven by professional interests and again this is an insight which helps to illuminate the British experience.[72]

Back at the London Clinic, how did it actually operate in its early years? Statistical data is fragmentary, but it seems that from the outset the institution dealt with significant numbers of children. So, for instance, in the second half of 1931 nearly 300 patients were referred with almost exact parity between the sexes. In 45 per cent of these cases 'the full resources of the Clinic, medical, psychological, and social were brought to bear on the case'. Another 45 per cent required only 'some simple form of treatment', with the remainder needing merely advice.[73] A report covering the period from the clinic's opening to the end of 1931, meanwhile, noted that the staff consisted of three psychiatrists plus Moodie, two psychologists and seven social workers. Between them they had carried out more than 10,000 interviews in 1931. The majority of patients had engaged in conduct distressing to others rather than themselves and most had more than one problem. The underlying aetiology was, in other words, complex, and the behavioural issues presented were symptoms not causes. In by now familiar terms the most 'powerful and universal' factor in maladjustment derived from 'the emotional forces arising out of the attitude adopted towards the child and towards his difficulties by other members of the family, by teachers, or, in fact, by anyone with whom he might be closely associated'. Treatment consisted primarily of advice to parents and it was 'fortunate' that problems were generally emotional rather than material in nature since it was easier to change parental attitudes than socio-economic circumstances. Much of this work was, of course, carried out by the PSWs. Finally, two postgraduate studentships in psychology and two in psychiatry had been founded by the Commonwealth Fund for training to be undertaken at the clinic.[74] More generally, Thomson observes that one consequence of child guidance's emergence in London was that 'problem children were less likely to be labelled as mentally defective and were often reclassified as suffering from emotional problems'.[75] This would have added to the number of patients seen by the London Clinic.

The London Clinic features prominently throughout this work although it will also be shown that child guidance was far from being simply a metropolitan phenomenon. Nonetheless it is equally worth noting that attention to its creation was not confined to Britain. So, for instance, in the US the National Council for Mental Hygiene sought information from the Commonwealth Fund in order to publicize developments in British child guidance. The same letter noted that a recent press release from the Federal Children's Bureau had included 'references to plans for the establishment of a child guidance clinic in London under the auspices of the Child Guidance Council'.[76] This further reinforces the argument that mental hygiene and child guidance were international concerns and that knowledge exchange and transfer were crucial components of their activities. We now turn to our final key development of the late 1920s, the creation of a training course for PSWs at the LSE.

The Diploma in Mental Health

The centrality of specially trained social workers to the child guidance project has been noted. Indeed Moodie was to argue in the early 1930s that the 'training of social workers is a more complicated matter than that of psychiatrists and psychologists, because the ground they have to cover is much newer to them and is wider in its scope' and that potential students should thus have a good academic and social work background.[77] We have also seen that British social workers had been sent to the US to observe child guidance practice and be trained in its techniques. Clearly, though, the latter process sought to provide a cohort of trained PSWs rather than constituting a long-term strategy. And so the Diploma in Mental Health course at the LSE came into being in 1929, located in the Department of Social Science and Administration.

This was preceded by another observational trip to the US early in 1928, apparently financed by the Commonwealth Fund, this time involving the LSE social work tutor Edith Eckhard. Her exhausting schedule included visits to the Boston Psychopathic Hospital, professional home of Adolf Meyer, the Cleveland Child Guidance Clinic, the Philadelphia Child Guidance Clinic and the National Committee for Mental Hygiene. On her return Eckhard wrote to Scoville that she had been 'much impressed' by the extent and thoroughness of the social work training she had observed, including in psychiatric social work. Eckhard added that she hoped to import some of the practices witnessed to the LSE and intended to insist that social work trainees had a Certificate in Social Science as a prerequisite for acceptance.[78] Presumably Eckhard's account was also circulated within her own institution. In any event, the issue of a dedicated course in psychiatric social work was raised by Fox with the School's director, William Beveridge, in late 1928. The latter, she reported to the Commonwealth Fund, had agreed to set up the course for three years provided the School did not incur any costs and provided he could get the approval of his professoriate and in particular Burt. Beveridge had been, Fox further commented, non-committal about what would happen thereafter.[79] Responding immediately, Barry Smith told Fox that the 'the training of psychiatric social workers is an essential and fundamental part of your child guidance program'.[80]

Shortly afterwards the CGC wrote to the Fund explaining why it had not sought any financial support for sending trainee social workers to the US. It was 'essential' to support the proposed new LSE course while simultaneously avoiding a situation whereby the best students were sent to New York. Training in New York should thus be reserved for those British social workers going on to hold 'special positions'.[81] On the same day the CGC also sent Beveridge what constituted a formal application to the School for the setting up of a 'one year course in Mental Welfare'. The letter noted that the Commonwealth Fund had allocated £400 per year for three years to the Council to be given in turn to the LSE to support running costs. Various proposals were made as to what might be included in the syllabus, what might be the entry requirements and the practical elements of the course in respect of work at clinics.[82] The actual content of the training is dealt with in the following chapter, but it is worth noting here that it was to be a matter in which various parties, including the Commonwealth Fund, felt they had a stake and an interest. For immediate purposes, though, what is important is the School's agreement with this suggestion and the decision to admit the first students later in the year.[83] This was the beginning of a more than decade-long, and often fractious, relationship between the LSE and the Fund.

From an administrative point of view the next important stage came in 1931 when the Commonwealth Fund and the CGC agreed that henceforth the financing of the Diploma should be taken out of the hands of the latter and dealt with directly by the Fund itself.[84] Beveridge, clearly a shrewd financial operator, continued to insist that the School could not itself put any money into the course now or in the future, a point emphasized in a letter to the Fund in March 1931.[85] But even before this Smith had told Scoville, in the wake of a meeting at the LSE, 'that Sir William Beveridge is a pirate of the first water, and he stuck out for every nickel he could get'.[86] Scoville appears to have concurred with this assessment of Beveridge's character, remarking later in 1931 that the School had 'deliberately "wangled" the budget for their own purposes'.[87] What was important, though, from the child guidance point of view, was that the Diploma had been established. This put in place training for a key group of workers in child guidance clinics and in the child patient's home. The foundations for spreading the child guidance message and carrying it out in practice were now in place.

Conclusion

This chapter has shown how and why child guidance came to Britain. As is already evident, this was a project which had particular aims to be promoted by particular professions and institutions. There were, again as is by now apparent, inconsistencies and tensions within child guidance and we shall see that these continue to raise crucial questions about the actual viability and coherence of the child guidance project. We next examine in more detail the three professions which constituted the child guidance team and the broader intellectual climate in which they operated.

2 PROFESSIONALS

Introduction

In the last chapter we saw how child guidance came to Britain, concluding with the setting up at the LSE of the Diploma in Mental Health. The latter sought to create a new profession, psychiatric social work. In turn this was part of a broader aspiration on the part of the Commonwealth Fund and the Child Guidance Council to promote a professionalized, even scientific, model of child guidance populated by three distinct professions and led by medicine – the American or medical model. This chapter examines the role of psychiatrists, psychologists and psychiatric social workers in the first decade of British child guidance, having first placed them in their broader intellectual context. The latter included claims to scientific status on behalf of both child guidance as a whole and on the part of each of the three professions. The American/medical model also wished to promote clinical teamwork in child guidance, but teamwork which was hierarchical. This was not, though, uncontested and claims to professional status and professional boundaries were important factors in driving forward, and giving shape to, British child guidance. Psychology, like psychiatry and psychiatric social work, was seeking to establish itself as a scientific and professional discipline and made claims to at least equality with psychiatry in child guidance practice. British child guidance, as was the case with child guidance elsewhere, was disputed territory.

Child Guidance and the Interwar Intellectual Climate

Before turning to the individual professions, however, we engage with the broader intellectual climate in which they operated, focusing on two particular issues: first, the social sciences and second, the physical world. It was a central plank of the European Enlightenment that human beings could employ reason and that with encouragement and education everyone would act rationally and thereby advance the cause of progress. Then there arrived thinkers such as Freud – the 'scientist of the mind' and a key contributor to the 'new psychology' – who argued that on the contrary, human behaviour is driven by a range of irrational and submerged impulses and forces. In Thomson's formulation what the 'new psychology' revealed was 'a mind with a mind of its own'.[1] By the 1920s there appeared to be more than sufficient evidence that reason was not being individually or collectively exerted. There was, for instance, the rise of avowedly irrationalist political movements such as fascism. And the First World War itself was increasingly seen as having served no purpose and as having achieved nothing – more irrationalism – and had also demonstrated, through the phenomenon of shell-shock, that otherwise normal men could under certain circumstances experience mental breakdown.

Such concerns were also present in other fields of social science. Currents in British interwar anthropology, for instance, sought to address problems of social pathology and maladaptation and were likewise influenced by the phenomenon of shell-shock. It is revealing to compare the remarks of Emanuel Miller on the problems engendered by civilization with those of W. R. Rivers, an influential contributor to both anthropology and psychology. Rivers, speaking in 1919, attributed the 'frequency of psycho-neuroses' in modern societies to the 'fluid and unorganized character of their civilization'. The 'perfect social organisation', he continued, was one in which 'instinctive tendencies, out of harmony with social ideals, have so come under control that they no longer form the grounds of conflict or give occasion for it only in the presence of exceptional stress and strain'. It is noticeable that Burt came into Rivers's sphere of influence and that Bowlby was influenced by him as an undergraduate, part of his more general interest in anthropology.[2]

Auden, in a discussion of the 'maladjusted child' and the consequent importance of child guidance, approvingly cited Rivers's work, remarking that primitive man was 'but ill-equipped by strength and agility for the struggle for existence'. Only through social organization was he able to survive. So while the infant child was 'essentially individualist' from birth he was 'subjected to a ceaseless stream of suggestions of social import from his immediate environment'. The child's mental make-up consisted at this stage of 'still plastic material' and it was this 'inherent suggestibility which gives to environment its supreme significance'.[3]

Sybil Clement Brown, meanwhile, recalled that in 1935, when she was course tutor on the Diploma in Mental Health, a 'discussion group including anthropologists, psychologists, sociologists, and psychiatric social workers' was organized at the LSE. This took as its starting point 'the conflict between adolescents and their parents which is widely prevalent in European societies'. Initially the social workers assumed that such conflict was 'largely due to the physical and psychological changes' associated with adolescence. This view, though, was 'considerably modified' when the relationship between adolescents and their parents 'in certain primitive societies', and where no such conflict took place, was described. Attention was thus shifted to the 'social phenomena of our society' wherein 'adult responsibilities are conferred relatively late and codes of behaviour are far less clearly defined'. The outcome was that 'the authority of parents tends to express itself in personal interference of a more emotional character than seems to be usual in simpler cultures'.[4]

This discussion group was, of course, located in the academic home of the leading British anthropologist of the interwar era, Bronislaw Malinowski, whose functionalist anthropology had supplanted that of Rivers. It is further notable that Bowlby later worked with one of the foremost anthropologists of her generation, who had through her fieldwork posed comparative questions about adult–adolescent relationships in primitive and advance societies, Margaret Mead. Child guidance practitioners were thus clearly aware of, and influenced by, aspects of contemporary anthropological thought, albeit in an eclectic and pragmatic way. Brown's concern with over-emotional responses in modern parenting, for example, had clear child guidance implications. And we shall presently encounter a child guidance practitioner later to become prominent in British anthropology.

Our second point about the intellectual context concerns the new understanding of the physical world and its broader cultural impact. The Newtonian world view whereby everything was ordered, stable and worked according to predictable laws – the physical world as a machine – was challenged by, for instance, the discoveries of quantum physics. Such new theories and hypotheses seemed to show a universe much less predictable and stable than had previously been understood. The psychiatrist Bernard Hart, one of the delegation sent to study American child guidance in the 1920s, told a professional audience in the early 1930s that developments in physics and mathematics had resulted in 'the concepts of causation and determinism [being] dethroned from their formerly unquestioned supremacy'.[5] What is especially notable here is that, as we shall see shortly, a few weeks earlier Hart had again addressed his professional colleagues, this time on maladjusted children and the child guidance clinics. And, assessing the impact of new theories in physics on psychology, Thomson notes that approaches which looked for a fixed consciousness or which promoted a 'mechanistic sensationalist psychology' or 'a consciousness that was fixed in time or space' were undermined.[6]

This was a world, then, where maladjustment, instability, lack of integration and human action and behaviour driven by unconscious forces was not just confined to unhappy children or by national boundaries. Instability was also inherent in the physical world and, in an era of economic, social and political disruption, in the very fabric of human society. Child guidance must therefore be seen as a particular response to much wider cultural, social and intellectual unease struggling with modernity and civilization.[7] Richard Overy characterizes the interwar period as Britain's 'morbid age' and points to the 'medicalization of the language of crisis', an observation clearly applicable to the child guidance project. Overy also points to how widespread social unease was while reminding us that 'science provoked profound ambiguity and was popularly understood to do so'.[8]

Child Guidance and Science

Nonetheless, science did hold a high intellectual and cultural status and all three child guidance professions sought to promote the idea that child guidance of itself was scientific and that their own disciplinary and professional approaches and practices were likewise grounded in scientific knowledge and method.[9] Such claims were important for the achievement, consolidation or enhancement of professional status, for promoting the shift from moral to scientific explanations of children's behavioural problems and because it gave weight to the authority exerted by psychiatrists, psychologists and PSWs over children and their parents.

The interwar era was also a time when, Steve Sturdy and Roger Cooter argue, a model of science based on 'systematic and rational investigation of the underlying causes and processes of health and disease' came to dominate medicine 'primarily because of the cultural values and ideals' they were perceived to embody.[10] Such a search for, and understanding of, underlying causes rather than superficial symptoms was central to the child guidance approach. Echoing Sturdy and Cooter's argument, Christopher Lawrence emphasizes the importance of the interwar years for medicine's transformation. Science and scientific research were, moreover, crucial not just to medicine but also as the means for 'analysing social problems and providing solutions to them'. The era was also characterized, Lawrence continues, by 'the flow of medical practices' from America to Europe underpinned by the power and ambitions of American philanthropy.[11] Again, this analysis fits well with British child guidance's trajectory.

What, then, were the claims to scientific status of psychiatry, the lead profession in the American/medical model of child guidance? As Gerald Grob argues of American psychiatry, from the late nineteenth century the profession sought to embrace not only mental disorders but also the 'problems of everyday life'. This was to be realized by a move into preventive medicine – the sort of move we have seen articulated in the British context by Moodie. What was thus being sought was the 'reintegration of psychiatry into medicine' so allowing the former to 'share in the status and prestige enjoyed by the latter'. In particular psychiatrists, like other medical scientists, sought to 'identify the causes of disease and to develop appropriate interventions for acute illnesses'.[12] So, for instance, Meyer was, as Katherine Angel points out, crucial in creating a 'new professional role for psychiatrists' thereby facilitating their membership of the 'scientific and medical establishment'. This move to 'place psychiatry on a par with scientific medicine' was complemented by 'a more general change in society's conception of mental illness and psychiatry', especially post-1918.[13] Such developments should be placed in the context of contemporary legislation and policy. Kathleen Jones observes that the 'Mental Treatment Act 1930 represented a marked change from a legal to a medical perspective'. The preceding Royal Commission had taken a public health perspective on mental illness and as Jones further remarks the Act was 'strongly normative' and emphasized the use of non-stigmatizing, and medical, terms such as 'doctor' and 'patient'.[14] The medical model of child guidance was thus part of, and contributed to, a realignment of both professional ambitions and social attitudes.

Specifically regarding children Hendrick suggests that ambitions to create a 'science of childhood' had characterized the Child Study movement of the late nineteenth century and that this and factors such as William Healy's attempt to 'establish scientific methods of approach to delinquency' fed directly into British child guidance. Hendrick also, though, remarks on the particular significance of the interwar period. This was an era when, as a result of medical and psychological developments, the interrelationship of mind and body came to the fore. Influential clinicians sought, furthermore, to place childhood within the remit of preventive medicine. Child guidance, Hendrick argues, was central to all of these developments.[15]

It is not difficult to find claims to scientific status for child guidance from psychiatrists. Moodie noted in the mid-1930s that the London Clinic had initially been viewed with considerable scepticism. This had changed, though, as a result of 'thorough, unobtrusive and scientific practice'.[16] Bowlby, utilizing material gathered at the London Clinic to analyse the origins of neuroses and the neurotic character, stressed the necessity of such studies and their importance for clinical work. It was, he continued, 'as important for analysts to make a scientific study of early environment' as it was for 'the nurseryman to make a scientific study of soil and atmosphere'.[17] Hart, in the child guidance speech alluded to above, claimed that the diagnosis and treatment of maladjusted or difficult children had shifted from 'an ethical to a physical conception, and thence to one predominantly psychological and biological'. Childhood's mental and emotional problems did not, therefore, derive from 'original sin' or exclusively from 'disease or disordered functioning of one or other organic system'. Rather, it was necessary to start with 'the conception of the child as a psycho-physical organism' whose mental or emotional equilibrium might be disturbed by a range and mix of environmental factors in combination.[18] Hart's speech again illustrates the shift from moral to scientific explanations for behavioural problems in childhood in the context of broader changes in psychiatry itself.

But psychologists and PSWs too claimed to be part of this scientific project. The psychologists James Drever and Margaret Drummond in discussing child guidance clinics rejected the idea that infants should not be the 'subject for scientific consideration and analysis'. The great majority of those attending such clinics, moreover, did not need medical attention. Rather, they were 'cases which demand psychological insight and a knowledge of modern psychological methods'.[19] The leading Scottish educationalist William Boyd told an audience in

1929 that the recently created Child Guidance Council was 'working on wrong lines because it regarded all sorts of maladjustments as problems for the psychiatrist'. Like Drever, Boyd argued that the majority of problems confronting both parents and teachers were educational 'in respect of both diagnosis and treatment'. Properly trained teachers – and the context here is that Scottish teacher training was to the fore in promoting educational psychology – could thus 'make a scientific use of mental and achievement tests' and so uncover 'maladjustments in the making'.[20] And as Boyd would later put it, at his Glasgow University clinic its 'clinicians were teachers versed in psychology'.[21]

The employment of clinical vocabulary reveals both psychology's aspiration to deal with the maladjusted child and its rejection of the medical model in favour of one based on psychological science. The former can also be seen as part of a broader process whereby psychology sought to establish its own scientific identity and to claim, as Rose puts it, a 'social role' which included the 'psychological discipline of the normal individual'. Dealing with 'maladjustment' and engaging with 'pedagogy and child rearing', he continues, were means of occupying this intellectual territory with the ultimate aim of a psychological science 'engineering the human soul'.[22]

Turning to PSWs, an American account of the profession's development helps illuminate the British experience. Sarah Swift reviewed the role played by the Institute for Child Guidance in New York, one of the locations for the training of the first cohort of British psychiatric social workers. She stressed the maturing of the profession to the point where the 'integration of psychiatric theory with practice achieved in handling the client relationship' advanced the PSW's role from that of a 'somewhat detached auxiliary' to the psychiatrist to 'one of greater responsibility and creative opportunity' – in other words, to a clinical role in diagnosis and treatment. The relationship between psychiatry and psychiatric social work was thus drawing ever closer, with the 'line of demarcation between the two' becoming 'less clearly defined'.[23] Here, then, was an ambitious claim for the profession. Its scientific basis was spelled out at a social work conference in Chicago in the early 1930s. Commenting on a case study presented by a social worker from the Institute for Child Guidance, a delegate remarked on the presenter's 'objectivity' and how this signified 'a scientific study of the problem rather than an emotional response to it'.[24]

This approach was shared by a number of British psychiatric social workers. Hunnybun, addressing a child guidance conference in 1935, observed that initially in Britain, as in the US, the PSW's role had been seen as a 'sort of lay assistant to the psychiatrist'. Now, however, she was engaged in more ambitious work which 'takes an active share in the plan of treatment, on a psycho-therapeutic level'.[25] Endorsing the need for an objective approach, Tilda Goldberg told another conference that the psychiatric social worker's role was that of interpreter, the central element of which was an 'approach towards human behaviour which characterizes all psychiatric treatment'. This entailed an 'attempt to understand and where necessary to change human behaviour by enquiring into its causes rather than judging it according to irrational and conventional standards'.[26] Such rejections of irrational or emotional responses to problems in childhood in favour of an objective, scientific approach are a yet further articulation of the need to replace moral explanations of childhood behaviours with psychobiological analyses. Goldberg, one of a number of refugees who took the Diploma in Mental Health, had studied psychology and economics at Berlin University before fleeing Nazi Germany in 1933. Qualifying as a PSW at the LSE in 1936, her first job was at a child guidance clinic in Hertfordshire.[27]

Revealingly, psychiatrists were at pains to stress the scientific nature of psychiatric social work. Moodie, for instance, suggested that the investigation of the child's home was 'no matter of question and answer, but of scientific observation', essential if accurate information was to be fed by the PSW into case conferences. Moodie further added that 'extremely scientific observation of the home environment' was necessary since it was 'impossible to assess a child's reaction to that environment, unless we have a clear picture of the emotional forces existing therein'.[28] R. G. Gordon, meanwhile, claimed that the specially trained PSW was essential to child guidance not least because she could thereby 'avoid the pitfalls with which the path of the well-meaning "common-sense" worker is so liberally strewn'.[29] Professional, scientific social work therefore eschewed both moral and casually empiricist accounts of childhood problems.

A note of caution, though, needs to be sounded. Elizabeth Lunbeck in her discussion of American psychiatry notes that in the 1920s PSWs adopted 'psychotherapy as a technique, establishing thereby a more theoretically consistent and scientifically derived conception of casework'. This had been partly generated by the 'resentment and anger' deriving from 'constant skirmishes' with psychiatrists dismissive of their training and who saw social workers primarily as their auxiliaries. The claim to scientific status by PSWs was therefore part of their attempt to present themselves as fellow professionals and not subordinates.[30] We are thus alerted to the possibility that similar issues may have emerged, for as we shall presently see, scientific or not, psychiatric social work was for British psychiatrists always under their own ultimate direction.

Whatever the reasons, there can be little doubt that PSWs saw themselves as distinct from, and more professional than, more traditional social workers and that this distinction was based on purportedly scientific knowledge and practice. This claim to scientific status was shared by psychiatrists and psychologists although in the case of all three professions there is a rather uneasy sense of the claim always having to be justified. Of course none of this was unproblematic and further suggests tensions between the three professions involved in child guidance. To engage more fully with these issues we now examine more closely their respective roles.

Psychiatrists

In the introductory chapter we encountered the psychiatrist Dr Barton Hall, who stressed the centrality of the 'science of medicine' to child guidance. Unsurprisingly, this was a view widely shared by fellow doctors and psychiatrists. Moodie, in a letter to the *BMJ*, remarked that: 'Child guidance clinics are controlled by a medical director, who, besides being skilled in the general practice of medicine, has a specialized knowledge of the uses and limitations of the various departments under his control'.[31] Henderson similarly argued, in a lecture to professional colleagues, that no patient attending a child guidance clinic 'showing defect or abnormality of behaviour or lack of social adaptation has been satisfactorily examined unless a complete medical and psychiatric examination has been made'. 'Psychologists and educationalists', he continued, 'are developing the habit of saying that this or that is "not medical", but either purely psychological or educational, and they do not hesitate to embark on psychopathological investigations, and even treat patients. There is danger here'.[32] The need for the appropriate training of the medical profession, meanwhile, was highlighted by Miller and Burke. No practitioner should attempt child guidance work without a 'thorough and practical grounding in both general and psychological medicine'. This required a 'lengthy medico-psychological training' without which there would develop a 'superficiality in outlook against which this new department of medicine must be safeguarded'.[33]

None of this meant that teamwork was unimportant – indeed Moodie published a pamphlet on the subject in which he argued that previously the fundamental causes of children's behavioural problems had been poorly understood. One outcome was that 'Child Guidance by team work has, therefore, been evolved so as to offer a more effective method of investigation than that used in the past'. Moodie further conceded that there were necessary tasks, such as measuring intelligence and making home visits, for which psychiatrists were either not equipped or did not have sufficient time. These could be better or more efficiently carried out by psychologists and PSWs. Nonetheless, the clinic's work was 'primarily psychiatric' so that, for instance, with regard to treatment the psychiatrist was the 'lead figure'.[34] In short, child guidance was a further instance of the 'hierarchical teamwork' identified by Sturdy and Cooter who also point to the push to organize medicine around the principles of scientific management.[35] This fits well with the child guidance case not only in terms of hierarchical division of labour and clinic organization but also through, for instance, systematic observation and record-keeping.[36]

But in broad terms what kind of approach did psychiatrists adopt? In 1927 the Secretary of the Charity Organization Society wrote to the Board of Education commending the emergence of British child guidance. It was possible, he wrote, that 'the idea of child guidance might suggest psycho-analysis and other psychiatric devices which do not command universal confidence' as well as being 'too new to expect a complete recognition from a great public authority' like the Board. In his view, though, the work carried out in America under Commonwealth Fund guidance was of a 'solid and conservative character'. Help for maladjusted children consisted of 'patience, sympathy, and concentration of ... experienced workers upon each child over a considerable period of time'. His organization was a long-standing advocate of such case work and supported the present Commonwealth Fund proposals.[37] These were very shrewd observations which again raise fundamental questions about what child guidance was, what it sought to achieve, and how – the idea that it was essentially social case work is especially revealing. For present purposes, though, we concentrate on the remarks about psychiatry.

It is difficult to generalize about the type of psychiatry employed in child guidance clinics partly because of the nature of the remaining case records, partly because of the eclectic nature of practitioners and practice and partly because it was, in any event, the PSWs who were most engaged in day-to-day work. But issues were certainly identified by contemporaries. The Feversham Committee, which investigated the voluntary mental health services in the mid-1930s, observed that in child guidance the 'psychiatric, or more strictly medical, aspect' showed a 'less well-defined course of development' than psychology or psychiatric social work. Moreover, many of the cases presently handled by clinics were 'so straightforward that psychiatric treatment is unnecessary' and would in time be dealt with by parents, teachers and other social agencies under the supervision of general practitioners (GPs) with only the more complex receiving psychiatric attention.[38] This comes close to denying altogether psychiatry's relevance.

Even someone as committed to psychiatrically led child guidance as Mac-Calman conceded that the 'therapeutic methods used by psychiatrists vary according to their personal capabilities, interests, and theoretical outlook'. Treatment was certainly based on a 'sound knowledge of psychopathology' but given the present state of knowledge 'remains ... very much an art in which success depends on the skill with which the therapist uses his personal contact with the child'. The imperfect understanding of 'behaviour and personality difficulties' further meant that specific 'therapeutic measures and techniques' were 'still a matter of theory and conjecture'.[39] This concern over the weakness of psychiatric knowledge about child development, and the associated problem of the training of psychiatrists, were issues to which MacCalman repeatedly returned. In short, the relatively small number of psychiatrists working in child guidance was acting in different ways in different places and on the basis of limited understanding.

But it is nonetheless possible to build up at least a partial picture of what psychiatrists claimed they were doing, and equally importantly, not doing. We begin with the latter. A report on the London Clinic compiled in the mid-1930s claimed that on its foundation it was seen as 'imported from America' and linked with psychology (by which was meant psychological medicine or psychiatry) with its 'very unwholesome associations in the public mind'. So, for instance, it had been suggested that 'children would be psychoanalysed against their parents' will' with one newspaper article making this claim with the headline 'Psycho-absurdity'. Consequently, the clinic's early demise was widely predicted.[40] Burke, while far from hostile to psychoanalysis per se, noted that at the East London Clinic to 'practise this method … would be folly' given the level of public scepticism. Clinics were, moreover, not organized in such a way that psychoanalysis could take place, it was debatable whether psychoanalysis was applicable to children and, in any event, neither he nor Miller were psychoanalysts.[41] Miller himself, recalling child guidance's early days, claimed that while the work of Susan Isaacs had gone some way to breaking down barriers, nonetheless 'any fraternizing between psycho-analysts and child guidance was not encouraged'. At this point there was, he continued, a 'tendency, fortunately short-lived, to dichotomize individual deep therapy and environmental manipulation'.[42] Miller did not indicate when he thought this dichotomy resolved although his remark flags up some future trends in child psychiatry.

Edward Mapother, psychiatrist at the Maudsley Hospital in London, wrote to the Commonwealth Fund in 1930. He noted that there could be resistance to child guidance because there was a 'marked tendency to suspicion of what is vaguely called Psycho-analysis of the Child, meaning detailed psychological investigation, and perhaps particularly such investigation of sexual matters'. Mapother continued that he had heard it said that 'the party of suspicion is largely a Roman Catholic one, that "Psycho-analysis" is regarded as poaching on the preserve of the Confessional'.[43] Strange as this might sound, it had some substance, although concerns about psychoanalysis were not confined to any particular religious group.

Moodie in particular was anxious to dispel any idea that psychoanalysis was a common psychiatric tool or even employed at all. In 1931 he wrote in a teachers' journal that in child guidance 'psycho-analysis is not used, but rather informal discussions of specific fears, obsessions, ceremonials and so on'. When treating children the crucial context was that 'injudicious investigation into their mental workings may be extremely harmful'. And given that many children's behavioural problems derived from their environment then 'the best thing to do is to leave the child alone and to straighten out the environment as far as this is possible'.[44] In a further review of the London Clinic in the mid-1930s Moodie again categorically stated that: 'No attempt is ever made to alter the personality by psycho-analysis'.[45] The only minor concession Moodie appears to have been prepared to make, although it had to do with treatment rather than diagnosis, was when he noted that little use was made of 'direct psycho-therapeutic treatment of an intense nature' because 'temperamental disturbances of a pathological nature' were rare – the point being that it was not ruled out completely.[46] Moodie's position is strange given that Bonnie Evans and her colleagues find that when at the Maudsley he had utilized psychoanalytic theory in treating very young children, albeit 'simplified psychoanalytic theory'.[47] What is clear, though, is that by his child guidance days he was keen to portray a particular image of his new project.

The rejection of psychoanalysis in child guidance was part of a wider social and cultural ambiguity in post-1918 Britain. Graham Richards suggests that it was certainly the case that in the 'fraught postwar context ... psychoanalysis initially found a receptive ... audience'. Similarly, a number of works dealing with childhood had significant psychoanalytical input and psychoanalytic language had begun to be embedded in popular discourse. On the other hand there were undoubtedly areas, not least sexuality, where 'cultural resistance' took place.[48] Thomson points out the medical profession's early opposition to Freudianism. This had to some degree broken down by the late 1930s – the BMA set up a section on psychological medicine in 1937 – although it would appear that this had as much to do with medicine seeking to stake a claim on the field of psychology in general as to any adherence to strict Freudian principles and techniques. Indeed such a development was perfectly compatible with a mental hygiene approach, not least given contemporary concerns about the extent of mental ill-health in the population.[49]

Of course it is important here to acknowledge MacCalman's point about the diversity of approach, one implication of which is that some child guidance practitioners, albeit a very few, may have operated in a manner which at least sought to engage with analytic theory and practice. Bowlby's child guidance work fed into, for example, his psychoanalytically informed research into the causes of war.[50] In a further, intriguing, 'theoretical' twist, Mary Burbury of the Manchester Child Guidance Clinic sought to have the University of Manchester invite Carl Jung to give a lecture although it is not clear whether this actually took place.[51] Bowlby's research projects and the undoubtedly more broadly based interest in the analytical approach notwithstanding, though, British child guidance was wary of full-scale engagement with what were seen as controversial theory and practices.

But if psychoanalysis was largely rejected, what approach was taken? A useful starting point here is, once again, Meyer and especially Edward Shorter's critique. Shorter finds Meyer a 'second-rate thinker' prone to adopting whatever new approach came along.[52] Leaving aside his intellectual capacities it could still be argued that what characterized Meyer's approach was eclecticism and pragmatism. This, of course, needs also to be seen alongside his insistence that the patient, including the child patient, be viewed as a psychobiological whole shaped not just by mental processes but also by environment.[53] Given Meyer's influence on British child guidance and psychiatry generally, and what we have seen as the anxiety of practitioners such as Moodie to dispel fears about psychoanalysis, some sense of what the team's medical member engaged in starts to emerge.

As British child guidance began to establish itself, Moodie argued that it was 'essential that investigation of the child mind be carried out without his being aware of it'. Any attention drawn to the patient's 'own mental working' would result in 'an incalculable amount of harm' being done, harm which was possibly 'irremediable'. On the other hand it was 'quite possible for the skilled observer to obtain all the information he requires from one or two informal conversations with the child – without ever asking a leading question or making a suggestion'.[54] And in another publication in which he again stressed that 'psycho-analytic method is never employed in a Child Guidance Clinic', Moodie went on to observe that any child requiring 'mental treatment is always extremely conscious of, and acutely worried by his own abnormal thoughts' and was thus ready to discuss them with a trustworthy adult, in this case the psychiatrist. Such a discussion, Moodie continued, 'need only follow the lines of an ordinary commonsense conversation' and indeed was 'all that is required. In the great majority of cases, no discussion of the child's thoughts is necessary or advisable'.[55] The notion of 'common sense', it is worth noting, was one often attributed to Meyer's approach.[56] As such it sits rather uneasily with the purportedly scientific claims described above as well as with the dismissal of the 'commonsense' social worker.

A straightforward technique was also extolled by the CGC. Its 1933 annual report observed that the 'methods employed are simple and straightforward, and have stood the test of time and of critical examination'. 'The general principle', it continued, was 'to use the simplest possible procedure which will attain the desired results'. In some cases 'simple advice' to a parent or teacher was all that was required. Unsurprisingly, the 'psycho-analytic is not applied'.[57] Illustrating the wider impact child guidance was now beginning to have, these passages were approvingly cited by the Board of Education's CMO.[58]

The Commonwealth Fund, meanwhile, remarked in the mid-1930s on the notable expansion in the number of British clinics. This was due in part to the London Clinic's 'careful and conservative' work. The word 'conservative', the report continued, was used advisedly. In the late 1920s proponents of British child guidance 'were sufficiently impressed by American precedents' to invite Fund support. But clinics were slow to develop until, inter alia, 'they had become well rooted in the traditions of British psychiatry'. The report then cited a statement by the London Clinic's staff which argued that:

> In comparatively new work such as child guidance, there is always a tendency to cultivate methods based on spectacular and attractive theory, and to develop new approaches before the old ones need to be discarded. The principle in the Clinic is to advance slowly and carefully, always on the firm foundation of experience, even though this may at times seem dull.[59]

The implied contrast here is with American child guidance, purportedly more psychoanalytically inclined or informed.[60]

In summary, the psychiatry employed in British child guidance was at best pragmatic, and at worst confused about what it actually sought to achieve and was in any event subject to variation between clinics and individual clinicians. Psychoanalysis was explicitly rejected in favour of the 'conservative' and 'common sense'. Child guidance psychiatry was acknowledged by proponents such as MacCalman as well as by the more sceptical Feversham Committee as being less well developed than other professional practice. Nonetheless, at least in England, psychiatrists were for the most part the lead figures in the interwar era, again evidence of the status ascribed to scientific medicine as well as of psychiatry's ambitions to be construed as such. Where, then, did this leave psychology and psychiatric social work?

Psychologists

As we have seen, child guidance psychologists too sought to establish their scientific credentials and to advance their professional status. A notable milestone here was the setting up in 1931 of the *British Journal of Educational Psychology* by the BPS. The journal's editor was C. W. Valentine, Professor of Education at the University of Birmingham and active member of the BPS's Birmingham branch, while the editorial board included prominent figures such as Burt, Drever and Spearman.[61] This publication was to provide a platform for debates about psychologists' approaches to child guidance and the standing of their profession vis-à-vis psychiatry. And it was certainly the case that developments in psychology – and particularly the psychology of individual differences – were seen as invaluable to child guidance. So, for instance, a recommended reading list on child psychology, published by the CGC and devised by a team including the psychiatrist Miller and the psychologist Fildes, listed works by leading psychologists such as Burt, Drever, William McDougall and the American behaviourist J. B. Watson as well as psychiatrically based readings by Sigmund Freud and R. D. Gillespie.[62]

What, though, did psychologists actually do? Psychometric testing was the bedrock of their child guidance function. The Oxford clinic utilized a system based on the Binet–Simon scheme and noted that it had been drawn up in such a way as to reduce by a 'very considerable degree' the influence of the 'personal element on the part of the examiner' – more evidence of the search for scientific objectivity. Children were asked, for example, to memorize sequences of numbers and to repeat sentences spoken by the psychologist. Marks were given accordingly and when completed this allowed for the calculation of the child's intellectual age.[63] The East London Clinic recorded that it had adopted and developed a number of verbal and non-verbal intelligence tests. It too used the revised, English, Binet–Simon scheme in 'conformity with the tradition prevailing in clinical psychology'. Tests of temperament and personality had been tried but ultimately rejected as '[m]uch more can be learnt about the temperamental and personality qualities of a child by careful clinical observation of its behaviour in the ordinary performance test situations'. In this particular clinic such observation was carried out by both the psychiatrist – Miller – and the psychologist – Dr Meyer Fortes. For pre-school children, meanwhile, the Merrill–Palmer scale had been adopted and, again, insights into the infant's personality could be gained by 'clinical observation of his spontaneous reaction' to these materials. Such traits as 'over-dependence, distractibility, negativism' were 'self-evident'. The average IQ score was 97. The clinic was 'thus dealing with what seems to be a fair sample of the child of average intellectual ability'.[64]

Fortes, later Professor of Anthropology at Cambridge University and thus an embodiment of the point made above about child guidance and anthropology, had done doctoral research at University College London with Spearman and had gained a Ratan Tata research studentship at the LSE for his work with Miller.[65] Fortes's career trajectory was thus rather unusual in child guidance (or any other) terms. Having said that, his entry to the field is indicative of the range of backgrounds, experiences and skills found in his co-workers. As a new area of medical, social scientific and social endeavour and one in which the professions concerned were either trying to establish or reinvent themselves, this is not altogether surprising.

In an article in *Mother and Child* Fortes gave an illuminating account of his child guidance work. He started by pointing to advances in psychological understanding and in particular regarding individual difference. What he described as 'Effective Intelligence' had, he argued, a number of different components which were not necessarily evident even to trained professionals such as teachers. For 'scientific and ... child guidance purposes' it was necessary to distinguish between these and to take them into account in treatment so that the difficult child could learn how to properly adapt to his environment. The psychologist thus sought to discover whether the child had 'enough native capacity to meet the demands of his environment, and what special abilities or disabilities, over and above this, he has'. Administering intelligence tests and the simultaneous observation of the child were how the psychologist reached his conclusions. As well as the Binet test, which was for the most part verbal, more 'concrete' activities were set, for instance jigsaw puzzles. To illustrate his point Fortes cited the case of a girl of high intelligence who was nonetheless poor at arithmetic. 'Superficially', he remarked, 'she seemed merely stupid at arithmetic'. However, the 'qualitative study of how she handled arithmetical problems showed ... that this stupidity was merely a symptom of a remote disturbance which had to be set right before any progress was to be expected of her in arithmetic'.[66] This case is revealing not only in terms of the techniques employed but also in highlighting psychologists' clinical aspirations. No doubt in this particular instance it was the psychiatrist who unearthed the 'remote disturbance'. But, equally, it was Fortes's initial measurements and observations which cleared the path for full diagnosis and treatment.

Other psychologists were especially forthright in asserting their profession's clinical claims underpinned by scepticism about maladjustment as primarily a medical issue. In 1935 Drever told a conference that the essence of child guidance was certainly teamwork. But the idea that psychologists be confined to mental testing was 'palpably absurd' as was any restriction of their role to 'the intellectual aspect of the child's mental life'. Failure to recognize a broader clinical responsibility would lead to the creation of separate psychiatric and psychological clinics, to the detriment of both.[67] In a book published the following year, Drever and his co-author again noted that teamwork was one of child guidance's key features and indeed had probably been 'one of the most valuable of the contributions which the movement has made to social service'. Medical, psychological, social and educational insights were all necessary. Hence the team required experts in all of these fields – that is, 'an expert in children's diseases, a psychologist, a director of social enquiries, and a specially trained teacher'. The psychiatrist, in other words, should be supplanted by a paediatrician and an educationalist added to the team. It was no doubt with such needs in mind that it was also suggested that going by the British experience 'we must interpret "child guidance" much more widely ... than the original intention even of the Child Guidance movement would lead us to suppose'.[68]

Boyd, meanwhile, later claimed in his unpublished autobiography that it was he who had set up the first British child guidance clinic in 1926, something 'ignored or disputed in England'. He and his colleagues had run this from the Glasgow University Education Department with the cooperation of local teachers. Boyd was, as we have seen, sceptical about psychiatry and here noted that

we set going a distinctive system of guidance. In England guidance was largely under the doctors. There had been imported with the aid of Rockefeller [*sic*] grants a system like the Americans with a psychiatrist (knowing nothing about education and not very much about children), at the head, a psychologist who gave the necessary tests and social psychiatric worker to get home details and act as a kind of mental nurse.

His practice, he claimed, was both cheaper and more effective and it was one of his protégés who was to go on to set up the local authority child guidance system in Glasgow in the late 1930s.[69] Boyd's own clinic was described in 1937 as 'particularly concerned with the problems of learning and behaviour met with in home or school and it gives much attention to temperamental causes of educational and personal difficulties'.[70] Drever later recalled that Boyd's clinic had been refused recognition by the CGC precisely because of its lack of psychiatrist

– hence Boyd's remark that his work had been 'ignored or disputed' – and that he himself had set up a similar clinic in 1927 in the Psychology Department of Edinburgh University.[71]

With such forceful advocates as Boyd and Drever, why was it that child guidance, at least in England, was in the interwar era 'largely under the doctors' while in Scotland different circumstances prevailed? The answer here has two dimensions: the weakness of psychology as a discipline and profession in England and by contrast educational psychology's strength in Scotland. The latter is discussed in the next chapter. As to the former, Wooldridge points to how the 'struggling profession' of psychology was, in child guidance, frequently in conflict with psychiatry. Psychiatrists, he remarks, 'tended to look down on psychologists' while psychologists 'often found psychiatrists unbearably arrogant and intolerably ignorant of child development' – exactly the sort of criticisms made by Boyd and Drever. Crucially, as Wooldridge further argues, the 'Commonwealth Fund's grant played into the hands of psychiatrists and psychiatrically trained social workers' who 'extended their control over the movement during the 1930s', with psychologists being on occasion reduced to 'little more than mental testers'.[72] In the light of what we have encountered of at least some psychologists' clinical activities, this clearly needs to be moderated – but Wooldridge's analysis is, nonetheless, compelling.

John Hall similarly highlights psychology's weakness in England, noting the discipline's slow development particularly when compared with the US and Germany. He further notes that educational psychology had no 'nationally agreed training schemes or professional structures'.[73] Thomson remarks upon the limited impact of psychology as a discipline on child guidance although he makes the important point, which qualifies Hall's argument, that it had a much greater impact on pedagogy and thus had 'important supporters at the heart of the educational establishment'.[74] To this might be added the intellectual outlet and stimulus of the *British Journal of Educational Psychology*. It was by building upon such initially shaky foundations that psychology was to reassert itself in child guidance, ultimately with official backing.

Psychiatric Social Workers

But what of the third member of the child guidance team, the psychiatric social worker? The history of social work has until recently been the subject of historical neglect, a point forcibly made by David Burnham. Such work as has been done, he argues, tends to be 'Whiggish' in tone and to emphasize notions such as professionalization and the discontinuities of the 1940s when, purportedly, the advent of the welfare state inaugurated a fundamental shift in social work theory, organization and practice.[75] Recently, though, greater attention has been paid to what Chris Nottingham characterizes as 'insecure professionals' such as social workers.

Research undertaken by, most notably, Vicky Long has provided much greater insight into psychiatric social work.[76] Notwithstanding their deficiencies in other respects, and in particular being written from an 'insider's' point of view, there also exist valuable accounts by PSWs themselves of what it was they sought to do.[77]

Psychiatric social work emerged first in the US in the aftermath of the First World War with training being offered at Smith College and at institutions such as the Institute for Child Guidance in New York. In America, as subsequently in Britain, psychiatric social work was intimately tied up with the development of child guidance. As the official report on the training of mental health social workers (noted in the introductory chapter) further remarked, the LSE Diploma in Mental Health 'was part of a scheme for the establishment of a child guidance service in this country' with both underwritten by the Commonwealth Fund.[78] The LSE's role reminds us too of the visit paid to the US by leading British advocates of child guidance and the opportunities thereby to observe PSWs in operation, as well as of child guidance and mental hygiene's international dimensions. The last point is further witnessed by the presence in the interwar period on the LSE course of overseas students. The Diploma was, for example, recognized as a suitable training for Dutch social workers and in 1939 the student body included two Dutch, one South African and one Australian, with overseas numbers being further expanded by refugees from Germany and Czechoslovakia.[79]

As to numbers and background, an analysis of the Diploma's first decade showed that of the 179 students who had taken the course 70 had university degrees. It was a course requirement that students have a qualification in social science – around one third of the students had gained this at the LSE itself – and previous social work experience. The largest single destination for those awarded the Diploma (143 students) was child guidance clinics (37) closely followed by mental hospitals.[80] So as Richard Titmuss was later to recall, the course was 'designed for experienced social workers ... who wish to gain further understanding of the causes and treatment of personal difficulties and problems of behaviour in children and adults'. Titmuss also noted the course's international appeal and that many Diploma holders had gone on to teaching careers in British universities.[81] This in turn reminds us of the view, forcefully held by PSWs themselves, that this was a specialism of a new and advanced kind. As Jones comments of America, 'child guidance social work belonged to a new breed, with intellectual ties to dynamic psychiatry as well as roots in nineteenth century altruism'.[82] Burnham argues that in Britain the 'body of knowledge elite groups of social workers chose was psycho-social casework, as promoted by American writers such as Charlotte Towle'.[83] Towle was, in fact, more than just a writer. She was a Philadelphia social worker who sought to carve out a particular, clinically based niche for PSWs based on, for instance, the pathologizing of mothers who brought their children to child guidance clinics.[84] In short, PSWs viewed their work as being in the vanguard of social work theory and practice and consciously adopted approaches which they felt reinforced this claim.

It is thus revealing that the constitution of the Association of Psychiatric Social Workers (APSW) described its aims as embracing the promotion of mental hygiene, including by means of engagement with research, raising and maintaining professional standards and encouraging the employment of properly trained workers at an adequate salary.[85] This was an aspirational programme very much in line with a body striving to emphasize its professional credentials. Equally revealing is the APSW's choice of presidents, an honorary role which was held at various points by leading psychiatrists such as Hart and Bowlby and individuals prominent in social policy such as Titmuss.

What did training in psychiatric social work involve? Some sense of this can be gained from the first course syllabus, devised jointly by the CGC and the LSE. The course lasted one year with time split between attendance at academic lectures (two days per week) and practical placements at appropriate institutions (the London Clinic was to be one of these, and so recognized for PSW training). Students would take sixty hours of classes on a range of subjects. The single largest class, taking up seventeen hours, was on psychiatry, although the three branches of psychology dealt with – Individual, Social and Abnormal – together absorbed twenty-three hours. The psychiatry classes were to embrace, inter alia, 'Psychological foundations of abnormal mental states. The theories of Freud, Jung and Adler'; 'Psychiatry and its bearing on Family and Social Relations'; and 'Special Symptoms that Appear in Children ... Their importance, and their treatment'. Classes were also taken on various aspects of social work – although presumably because entrants had to have pre-entry social work experience this was kept fairly minimal – and the administration of hospitals and the Mental Deficiency Acts. The sessions on social casework included 'Child Guidance ... Genetic study of personality. The necessity for a complete picture. The fourfold study.[86] How a Clinic is organized to obtain this material. Essential unity of investigation and treatment'.[87]

This was clearly an ambitious course much in advance of other contemporary forms of social work training. But as the hours committed to the various topics and their very number already suggest, the depth in which these could be studied in a relatively short time is open to question. We return to this below. Nonetheless, students were exposed to key child guidance and social work practitioners and teachers as well as some of the leading scientists and social scientists of the period. These included the ubiquitous MacCalman, Fildes and Burt. The last of these was not, it would appear, popular with either students or colleagues. Moodie wrote to the Commonwealth Fund in 1934 that there were 'complaints about Dr Burt's lectures, that he is too vague and unpractical'. Burt was, Moodie suggested, focused on his writing to the neglect of his teaching and under such circumstances 'it will be easy for him to become vague because his mind is like that anyway'.[88] This casual insult could simply be a reflection of Moodie's personal feelings or could suggest scepticism about Burt's work and his influence on his fellow psychologists, one which Moodie was happy to share with Fund officials. From outside of child guidance, meanwhile, students could also attend lectures given by the criminologist Hermann Mannheim and the physician and specialist in mental defect Lionel Penrose.[89]

But the contributor to the Diploma course, and later its leader, on whom we particularly focus in order to illustrate further her profession's aims and aspirations, is Sybil Clement Brown. Brown had an increasingly high profile in social work and social policy circles. She also wrote for popular journals such as *Mother and Child* as well as for fellow professionals, most notably in a post-war work co-authored with another prominent PSW, Margaret Ashdown.[90] Brown was held in high regard by the Commonwealth Fund and one particular episode in their mutual relationship is revealing about how child guidance was viewed, not least from a social work angle, in the mid-1930s. In April 1934 Scoville told Barry Smith that during her recent visit to the LSE she had suggested that Brown come to the US. Brown had responded enthusiastically and Moodie too had been strongly in favour. However Noel Hunnybun, who had herself undertaken training in New York, had expressed doubts about such a visit on the basis that many of those involved in British child guidance 'were still sceptical of so much American influence'. Hence a trip to the US 'might create some prejudice against Miss Clement Brown'. Scoville was not convinced and sought Moodie's support. This she received, and Brown duly travelled in the summer of 1935.[91] What is immediately revealing is Hunnybun's concern over perceptions of American influence, which as we have seen was shared with others in British child guidance and which had been used by Fox as a means of attacking Hunnybun herself.[92] Uneasiness about undue American influence was clearly an ongoing issue.

Brown toured a number of psychiatric social work training centres and gave an account of her experiences. Placing her observations in the context of political developments such as the New Deal and thereby anticipating later historians who locate child guidance in progressive American social reform, she remarked that 'psychiatric social work pursues an admirably courageous if often a bewildered course'. It had survived attacks by its critics and 'more child guidance clinics opened last year than in any previous year'. There were professional differences of opinion but there were also 'signs of a desire to leave behind this adherence to schools of thought' – another, unwitting, indicator of child guidance's eclecticism and pragmatism – and 'to think instead in terms of particular treatment needs of individuals, the appropriate function of agencies, and the specific personal skills of students and workers'. Crucially, within training institutions there was thus 'far more stress upon the discussion of detailed methods of treatment than there is upon causation'.[93] In both America and Britain, in short, treatment was on the psychiatric social work agenda.

Brown was also, as we have seen, intellectually curious enough to engage with scholars from other disciplines. Moodie, in a letter to Scoville, remarked that 'Miss Clement Brown is at present in one of her phases of philosophical thought, and is for the time being more interested in the sociological implications of problem behaviour than in the child guidance case pure and simple'.[94] This was a shrewd observation as Brown was indeed keen to reflect on social work theory and methods. In an essay published in the late 1930s, and deriving in part from the inter-disciplinary LSE discussion group where she had encountered anthropologists and other social scientists, Brown laid out her views.

Social work's aim could be summarized 'as the promotion of a greater degree of compatibility between the needs and desires of the individual and the requirements of society'. Recently, a new branch – psychiatric social work – had emerged and PSWs collaborated with 'medical and educational psychologists' in studying and treating mental disturbance and delinquency and in promoting 'mental health through the "guidance" of children'. Brown had made a comparative analysis of case records from 1924 and 1934. In 1924, social workers' commentaries were primarily concerned with qualities such as 'honesty' and with material surroundings. There had been a shift, though, due to the 'growing conviction' that social problems were more dependent upon an individual's attitudes and intimate social relationships than upon 'superficial habits and physical surroundings'. Ultimately, the task of PSWs and other specialists was to decide which 'facts' were of especial significance to any given problem and to 'select that theory of interrelationship which seems to offer the most comprehensive explanation'. The 'scientific justification' for such an eclectic approach lay in the melding of practical experience with specialized knowledge. In child guidance 'the type of knowledge which leads to deductions as to aetiology and prognosis is seldom related to the causes of specific symptoms' not least because with respect to personality and social behaviour 'apparently similar situations may produce quite different results'. So with respect to 'prediction and treatment', what was most useful was an awareness of which family situations were apt to produce maladjustment and 'the nature of the responses characteristic of different types of personality'. Interest was consequently shifting from 'the content to the functions of maladjustment'. Hence while previously social workers had usually been 'called upon to deal with the symptoms of friction', it was 'only in recent years that a more positive aim can be discerned'.[95]

Burnham cites this essay as a further example of the influence of American theory and practice on elite British social workers such as Brown, perhaps thereby retrospectively justifying Hunnybun's concerns.[96] It was certainly a sophisticated and informed contribution making significant claims for psychiatric social work. This new branch of social work utilizes specialist knowledge and language and employs theories and methods which can be justified scientifically. It works alongside other professionals rather than in subordination to them, is concerned with individual psychology rather than material surroundings while nonetheless having a broader social mission and claims a role in the treatment of causes rather than the amelioration of their symptoms. Brown was undoubtedly a key figure in her profession who sought its advance not simply in terms of 'traditional' casework and treatment but rather through using a range of insights from a variety of disciplines. Her influence on both the LSE course and child guidance should not be underestimated. What is much more problematic is the extent to which her ideas actually informed day-to-day social work practice and the level of engagement which other PSWs and PSW students were able to bring to them.

There can be little doubt that many of the Diploma students derived considerable intellectual stimulus from such exposure. Nonetheless training in psychiatric social work does raise three important issues. The first is what did PSWs, once trained, actually do in practice? This is dealt with in more detail in chapter 4. In broad terms, though, it is argued that while on occasion PSWs based at child guidance clinics did indeed, in reporting their cases, utilize concepts derived from theoretical psychiatry and psychology, it was equally the case that much of their practical work was, in the last resort, 'traditional' social casework. And, various claims to the contrary notwithstanding, PSWs were not immune from employing moralistic language and judgements.

The second issue concerns the student body and, thereby, the profession. Psychiatric social workers claimed to be working alongside psychiatrists and psychologists rather than being subordinate to them. Given the professional self-perception of psychiatrists in particular this was, to say the least, rather implausible. Child guidance certainly involved teamwork but it was hierarchical teamwork, notwithstanding that it was PSWs who had most contact with children and their families. More than this, though, there was the gender composition of the three professions. Although there were a few exceptions the psychiatrists undertaking child guidance work were for the most part men as was the case with the medical profession in general. Psychologists, meanwhile, might be either male or female, a reflection, perhaps, of the opportunities available to women in a profession still trying to define itself. PSWs in child guidance, though, were in the interwar era without exception female. This was almost certainly taken for granted by those recruiting to the LSE course, a reflection of the prevailing view about who should enter the 'caring' professions. And given the nature of gender relations in Britain at this time (and for some time to come) then it was surely the case that the PSW's place in the hierarchical team was well and truly ensured.[97] As Jones pithily puts it, in the 'child guidance industry social workers became the work force, while psychiatrists were management'.[98]

The third issue relates to the course itself. There is no doubt that by and large it was seen in a positive light by the Commonwealth Fund, the LSE, the CGC and other interested parties. It was successful in attracting students, continued well into the post-war era and was until the 1940s the sole training centre for an increasingly in-demand profession. There were, however, also continuing tensions and debates about what was required of applicants, course content and duration and the balance between academic and practical work. The National Council for Mental Hygiene, for example, suggested in 1932 that while it welcomed the course's formation it also felt it to be 'too comprehensive, particularly on the theoretical side'.[99] Around the same time Barry Smith suggested to the LSE academic responsible for the course that for potential entrants previous social work experience was certainly highly desirable, as were academic qualifications. Nonetheless, it was his view that 'experience and personal qualifications are somewhat more important in this field than perhaps in some others'.[100] As to the placement encounter a report from those responsible for training PSWs at the London Clinic argued that: 'The period for practical work at the Clinic is far too short. It is felt that students who want to specialize in Child Guidance work should be here for at least a year'.[101] In 1937, meanwhile, a course on the 'Administration of Hospitals and Child Guidance Centres' had to be simplified as in its original form it had been deemed 'too advanced'.[102]

Perhaps most significant was a staff discussion which took place on the eve of the Second World War. This appears to have been engendered by a memorandum from Bowlby, on behalf of the teaching staff at the London Clinic, to which Burt and some of his colleagues took exception. The psychologist Lucy Fildes, for example, argued that she found 'difficulty in planning an adequate syllabus in the basic facts and concepts of psychology during this short course' and suggested that 'the teaching of speculative theories should be reduced rather than elaborated'. The latter comment is presumably a criticism of psychiatry while the former advances the claims of psychology. Other criticisms aired included that 'students did not appear at the present time to get from their psychology lectures knowledge which they needed for case work at the Child Guidance Clinic'. As a result of the war this debate reached no clear conclusion.[103] The structure and content of training in psychiatric social work continued to be an issue into the post-war era, with even enthusiasts such as Brown and her co-author admitting that it took place within 'the limits of a one year course'.[104]

Of course, all academic programmes are subject to debates and arguments about form and content and it would be wrong to be over-critical of the Diploma in Mental Health course on such grounds. Nonetheless the evidence cited does highlight, most notably, tensions between the academic and the practical in terms of balance and, given the duration of the course, concerns about both the academic depth possible and the utility of the practical experience. In turn, this raises more general issues about the role and status of PSWs.

Roy Lubove in his history of American social work poses the question as to how, ultimately, it is possible to distinguish between psychiatric social workers, psychiatrists and psychotherapists to which his answer is: 'the social worker's inferior training'.[105] Jones points out that in American child guidance, social workers were not able to 'generate professional autonomy or equality in the work place. Psychiatrists had earned a position of greater authority on the child guidance team'.[106] In short, hierarchical teamwork asserted itself and this was as true in Britain as it was in the United States. Contemporary gender relations and the nature of training in psychiatric social work played a major part in cementing this relationship. The content of training also, necessarily, had profound implications for what PSWs actually did with the clinic's child patients and their families and this in turn may be seen to seriously undermine the medical foundations on which child guidance, in England at least, claimed to be built.

None of this is to belittle the work of individual PSWs. It seems clear that, as we shall see in chapter 4, many did bring relief, at least of a practical kind, to children and their families at times of distress. Some, too, took the challenge of research seriously, producing important publications and papers. A notable example here is Robina Addis, who carried out an important investigation into bed-wetting, one of the main causes of referral to child guidance clinics.[107] And we have also noted the intellectual engagement of PSW leaders such as Brown in her mission to professionalize her occupation. But as Nottingham points out, such workers were 'messengers of obligation, witnesses to misfortune, administrators of society's zero sums'. Perhaps crucially, they 'rarely had much influence over the rules they applied though they could bend them'.[108] While hardly an unproblematic formulation this is nonetheless a useful way of conceiving those who were in the front line of child guidance while the recipients of what must ultimately be construed as a training which sought much but delivered less.

Conclusion

This chapter has examined the roles of the three professions engaged in child guidance work, particularly in the context of the idea of hierarchical teamwork. The medical model, promoted by interested parties such as the Commonwealth Fund, ascribed leadership to medically trained psychiatrists. PSWs and, in particular, psychologists challenged this without, at least in England, mounting a serious threat to hierarchical organization. What all three professions had in common, though, was their claim to scientific status both for their own work and for child guidance in general. This had three dimensions. First, science per se retained a high cultural and intellectual standing and was thus a desirable end in itself for such professions. In a world characterized by instability, moreover, scientific reason was to be used to counter the vagaries of the human unconscious and child maladjustment. Such an approach would, for instance, guard against extremes of emotion, extremes of any kind being a threat to individual, familial and social stability. Second, the scientific treatment of child maladjustment – carried out by specially trained professionals – was to be used to supplant preceding notions of moral explanations for behaviours deemed unacceptable or potentially risky. And, third, scientific expertise could be utilized to exert authority over patients, their families and the broader society. None of this was, though, unproblematic and issues around the PSW's role and the lack of clinical clarity and coherence employed by child guidance psychiatrists, not to mention psychology's rival claims, continued to be serious issues in British child guidance. We next look at its expansion in the 1930s.

3 THE SPREAD OF CHILD GUIDANCE
IN THE 1930s

Introduction

In this chapter we analyse the spread and dissemination of child guidance in the 1930s in three ways. First, we examine the propagation of child guidance ideas through various media and events. These included articles in popular journals and meetings for lay persons put on by child guidance staff. Note is also taken of the ways in which such staff sought to convert fellow professionals, non-medical and medical, not directly involved in this branch of child psychiatry and psychology. Second, we examine the spread of clinics to centres such as Liverpool, Birmingham, Manchester and Bristol (in 1930, 1931, 1933 and 1936 respectively, with Birmingham having a claim to be the first local authority clinic) and how this contributed to a wider acceptance of the child guide message in official circles. Third, we then turn to Scotland. Here, the Notre Dame Child Guidance Clinic in Glasgow was both an exemplar of the American/medical model and of a particularly Roman Catholic approach to child guidance. Scottish child guidance as a whole, though, was dominated not by psychiatry but by psychology, thereby sharply differentiating it from the predominant situation in England.

Publications and Talks

The idea that child guidance was about more than simply clinical work was to become especially pronounced after the Second World War. But in the 1930s, while still tending to emphasize the clinic's centrality, a concerted effort was made to promote the child guidance message to a much wider range of professional and lay audiences. This operated in a number of ways. In 1933, for example, Auden was invited by the BBC to make a radio broadcast on child guidance.[1] Miller later recalled that he, Moodie and Burt had all appeared on the BBC in 1932.[2] Their talks were later published in the popular BBC magazine the *Listener* and in a volume edited by Burt.[3] The CGC's annual report for 1938, meanwhile, noted that the 'demand for public enlightenment on child guidance and its kindred subjects' was growing as witnessed by requests for CGC pamphlets. 'Many thousands' had been distributed that year, 'especially at the Glasgow Exhibition' – that is, the Empire Exhibition. The Council also had its own increasingly popular travelling display which had now been shown in 'practically all large centres of population'.[4] All this points to a growing public interest in, and awareness of, child guidance as well as a desire on the part of practitioners to get their message across.

Another especially notable form of dissemination was by way of popular and didactic magazines and books. Peter Bowler has shown how such media were important in generally broadening the readership for scientific matters, reminding us also that child guidance had scientific pretensions.[5] Cathy Urwin and Elaine Sharland suggest that popular publications were an important mechanism in realizing the shift from body to mind in perceptions of children and childhood. More than this, though, they point to the 'transformation' which the interwar period brought to childcare literature and how this was 'linked to the unequivocal authority given to experts who based their advice on scientific principles'. Mothercraft, they continue, became 'a matter of national policy' and gained the support of the Board of Education's CMO, Sir George Newman.[6] All these points are borne out by child guidance.

So, for instance, Fildes and MacCalman were among the contributors to *Child Life*. The piece by the former was on 'Backwardness and Behaviour Problems' about which she concluded that 'backwardness' – which was not necessarily caused by intellectual shortcomings – could cause a child to be discontented since 'being itself the result of maladjustment, it intensifies the condition and leads to further maladjustment'. In such circumstances it was obvious that 'backwardness is a serious matter, and that children who suffer in this way should not be left to carry on as best they can, still less should they be blamed for their backwardness as if it were a sin'.[7] These were often-repeated points – that problems would not just go away of their own accord and what was at issue was not moral failing but emotional maladjustment. MacCalman addressed sleep disturbance. So-called insomnia was often, he claimed, 'but one of a number of behaviour difficulties which the child presents'. Such sleeplessness was 'really part of the spoiled child reaction, and there will be similar difficulties in feeding, dressing, and so on'. What was essential in all aspects of child management, he told readers, was 'regularity' and this pertained to sleep as much as to the establishment of good habits in other realms of the child's life.[8] The spoiled child was another child guidance preoccupation.

Of particular importance to the spread of the child guidance message to the educated lay public was the magazine *Mother and Child*, launched by the National Council for Maternity and Child Welfare in 1930 and published until 1974. It carried regular items about, for example, CGC activities and the opening of new clinics. In early 1939, for instance, it was noted that the East London

Clinic was relocating and that, in addition, local political disturbances had 'made the position of the clinic a matter of special concern to the community'. The clinic was, of course, a Jewish institution and the reference was to fascist, anti-Semitic, campaigning in the area. Fear and hatred had 'serious effects ... on a child's nervous system' and the problems such children were encountering had 'raised a new problem for the community'.[9] This was one of the relatively few instances where children's emotional and psychological problems were attributed to factors external to the child and its familial relationships or the more general circumstances of modernity.

The journal also regularly carried articles by leading child guidance practitioners focusing on particular problems or issues. So a series of eight lectures – public talks were another method of disseminating the message – on 'The Psychological Problems of Childhood' given at the Jewish clinic in 1932 were reproduced. These included Miller on 'The Mechanism of Behaviour Disorders and Psycho-Neurosis in Children' and the clinic's social worker, Beatrice Robinson, on child guidance's social dimensions.[10] Despite the rather forbidding title of Miller's piece these articles, like those cited from *Child Life*, were mostly written in non-technical and jargon-free language. Case studies were often used to illustrate the article's topic. The overall tone was didactic, clearly designed to offer parents (or more accurately mothers) advice on how to bring up their children, how to identify potential problems as early as possible and how thereby to avoid the 'mistakes' which the case studies appeared to demonstrate.

The authors' experience in clinics and as experts was thus what was being drawn upon while parental anxieties were being tapped into. More than this, parents were being encouraged to see their child's behaviour as potentially problematic and thereby as in need of surveillance and monitoring. Clinical approaches and lay concerns were thus in a symbiotic relationship with each feeding into and appearing to validate the other. More broadly, child guidance as explicated in such publications can be seen as exemplifying Ludmilla Jordanova's argument that 'the process whereby health and disease are conceptualized' involves many factors, including popular culture, advertising, art and literature, politics and policy-making.[11] Popular journals such as *Mother and Child* helped spread the child guidance message. As we shall see later in this and in the next chapter the number of child patients and the number of clinics rose throughout the 1930s. Of course professional interests were important here and many clinic referrals arose from professional intervention. But by no means all did and parental referrals were far from rare. This would suggest that child guidance's claims and ambitions were reaching beyond clinic workers or those in education or other social agencies.

But child guidance practitioners and supporters did also address audiences in professionally related fields and voluntary organizations with particular interests in child welfare. Moodie and MacCalman lectured on a course organized by the CGC for the Ministry of Health and aimed at those running children's homes and institutions. The lecture notes for this course covered issues such as emotional growth and development and argued for, inter alia, honesty about sex (children were less worried about this than adults), the need for discipline (too much freedom was in fact parental neglect) and the essentials for healthy mental development in children (security, affection, work and play).[12] Moodie, meanwhile, addressed a meeting at the Conference of Educational Associations in 1934 and a child guidance literature stall was also present at this event.[13] Two years later the CGC recorded that it had provided over 100 lectures, mostly grouped in specific courses, to organizations including the National Children's Home and Orphanage, a number of Teachers' Training Colleges, the National Council for Girls' Clubs and the National Council for Women in the North of England. The last of these resulted in a resolution for the general establishment of child guidance clinics being passed at the National Conference of the National Council of Women.[14]

Such growing public interest beyond professional concerns can also be found in the realm of politics. As we shall see, child guidance in the 1930s came to be increasingly driven forward by democratically elected local authorities – albeit often at the prompting of local medical staff, educationalists or philanthropists – and subsequently with the quiet encouragement of the Board of Education. But child maladjustment was being politically recognized in other ways. A Labour Party policy document from 1934 noted the existence of a 'considerable number' of maladjusted children. The average teacher could not be expected to 'deal with the problem, which is one for the expert physician or psychiatrist'. There were some clinics available to deal with such children including a few founded by local authorities. It was Labour's belief that 'centres of this kind should be much more common and that a competent staff of social workers, psychologists and medical men should be at their disposal'. The work of such clinics in diagnosing, treating and preventing maladjustment would thus 'bring science more fully to the service of education'.[15]

A few years later Labour published *A Children's Charter*, originally a report to the National Conference of Labour Women. In the section on child guidance it was suggested that the 'difficult' child could be found in most schools and that 'failure to understand and deal with him properly' might 'result in antisocial conduct during or after school years'. Difficulties arose from 'emotional disharmony and insecurity', generally the 'result of unfortunate home conditions'. Going off message, momentarily but predictably, the latter were often 'attributable to poverty'. So every LEA should have a child guidance clinic 'under the charge of medical and psychological experts'. The aid thus provided would 'reduce delinquency and save endless unhappiness and waste in later years'.[16] The adherence to the medical model is notable here as is the more general acceptance of the child guidance message.

And child guidance practitioners sought to keep their professional colleagues abreast of developments by way of articles and reports in publications such as the *BMJ* and the *British Journal of Educational Psychology* and through lectures and meetings. The *BMJ*, for instance, carried a report about a meeting on child guidance held at the Liverpool Medical Institution in 1933. One of those who spoke was the local clinic's psychiatrist, Dr Barton Hall, who suggested that identifying 'the causes underlying, and factors contributing to, childish fears, anxieties, obsessions, etc., in their early stages should do much to prevent the development of more chronic forms of neurosis in later life'. Such diagnosis and treatment could thus be seen as 'prophylactic'.[17]

Psychologists likewise sought to spread the message to their professional colleagues. Among the papers heard by the Society's Scottish branch in 1936 was one by the Glasgow psychologist Rex Knight on 'Child Guidance in Italy'.[18] Intriguingly, the *British Journal of Educational Psychology* carried not only articles by psychologists, as might be expected. It also took pieces by psychiatrists, for instance that by Miller on temperamental differences and behaviour problems in children, which was based on a speech to the Psychological Section of the British Association.[19] This professional generosity by psychologists to their medical colleagues appears to have been rarely reciprocated. Nonetheless, the journal's foundation and its members' activities indicate that the BPS was taking the issue of child psychology seriously and as such is a further indicator of broader professional, social and political concerns about the mental state of the nation's children.

There was, moreover, more to all this than simply information-sharing. Doctors and psychiatrists were also seeking to establish their credentials with fellow professionals, many of whom remained ignorant of, or hostile or indifferent to, psychiatric medicine – hence the relentless proselytizing of individuals such as Moodie. By the same token PSWs were interested in establishing their standing as leaders within social work through the formation of their own professional association and through a distinctive training course. This would further result in the setting up after the Second World War of the professional outlet the *British Journal of Psychiatric Social Work*. For psychologists, meanwhile, the issue was one of establishing professional status and in particular in a field, child guidance, to which they felt they had their own professional and clinical claims.

Clinics outside London

What, though, of the clinics to which these professionals were attached? We saw in chapter 1 that the founding of the London Clinic in 1929 had been a key moment in the establishment of British child guidance. The capital was to continue to be an important locale for child guidance services and in 1943 the LCC recorded eight recognized clinics within its boundaries, including its own at the Maudsley Hospital. The latter was the other location, besides the London Clinic, where student PSWs could receive practical training. The Council also noted its own support for child guidance from the outset and that this had included grants made to certain clinics, and especially the London Clinic.[20]

Before discussing the origins and developments of particular clinics outside London it is necessary to say something about the 'loan' system which the CGC provided for PSWs. In fact, this mechanism was also available to new clinics in London but its use was especially significant elsewhere because of the way in which it helped spread the child guidance message and practice. As a Commonwealth Fund report remarked, 'loaning' a PSW to a new clinic for one or two years 'was at once an indirect subsidy and a lever to establish the establishment of good standards'.[21] The 'indirect subsidy' was because the Council met the social worker's salary costs in the expectation that these would be taken up by the clinic or its supporters once it was soundly established. So, for instance, Birmingham's Education Committee noted in 1934 that the CGC had, with Fund approval, loaned a PSW to the local clinic 'for the two years ended 31st March 1934' and that it was now necessary 'to make arrangements for the continuance of [her] services'.[22] In 1938 MacCalman, by now attached to the University of Aberdeen, successfully applied for the loan of a PSW and was able to report the following year that the local authority and the university had now agreed to meet her salary costs.[23]

At its financial peak in 1934 the loan scheme constituted just over 25 per cent of CGC expenditure.[24] The subsequent decline in demand for such loans was, the Council suggested the following year, not attributable to 'any diminution in the demand for such workers'. On the contrary it was 'proof that the need for trained personnel is now recognised' by both statutory and voluntary agencies and these were thus 'prepared to make direct appointments without a preliminary trial period'. As we shall see, by this point the Board of Education had made a positive move in the field of child guidance finance. Such greater recognition notwithstanding the Council had still loaned social workers to clinics in Cardiff and Cheltenham.[25]

To return to Birmingham, its clinic was one of the most important outside London. Given his interest in and engagement with child guidance it seems likely that Auden would have been heavily involved in its development although no direct evidence exists. It was also more generally the case that Birmingham prided itself on its progressive reform agenda and that, as Ian Grosvenor and Kevin Myers point out, nowhere was this more so than in education. So, for example, the city was in the vanguard of provision for children with special needs.[26] Child guidance was first officially raised at a meeting of a subcommittee of the Corporation's Education Committee in late 1930.[27] As a historian of

Birmingham Corporation later noted, a clinic was duly set up in 1931 'for an experimental period of three years' and that financial support came from the Commonwealth Fund and an anonymous donor.[28] This support was crucial since at this point local authorities could not, in principle, spend money on such services. Olive Sampson, undoubtedly correctly, attributes the voluntary donation to Geraldine Cadbury, philanthropist and member of the important and influential Birmingham manufacturing family.[29]

The rationale for setting up a clinic was discussed at some length in a report presented to the Education Committee. This remarked, first, that the School Medical Service's present activities were inadequate or inappropriate for those children who were, in a further example of the range of behaviours deemed to signal maladjustment,

> intensely nervous or persistently shy or reserved ... unmanageable at school or at home, who appear to have tendencies to pilfering or dishonesty, who exhibit backwardness not due to intellectual retardation, or anomalies of speech development such as the persistence of baby speech, stammering or delayed speech, who have difficulty in controlling the natural functions of the body, and so on.

Various bodies, including the local branch of the National Union of Women, had urged the Corporation to take up child guidance, a further instance of the wider public demand for its services. Consequently the CGC had been approached and it was by this avenue that Commonwealth Fund support had been gained. It was also noted that the psychiatrist appointed would almost certainly gain a scholarship to study child guidance techniques and this indeed turned out to be so. All in all the monies deriving from the Fund and the anonymous donor would allow for the employment of a psychiatrist, a psychologist and a PSW for a maximum of three years 'without any cost to the rates'. When funding ran out the situation would be reviewed. All this was agreed to by the Committee.[30] Developments in Birmingham clearly impressed *Mother and Child* which commented that it provided an 'interesting example of the way in which the Child Guidance Council can help forward local movements'.[31]

The process of appointing a Medical Director appears to have taken longer than anticipated, but in autumn 1931 Dr Charles Burns was given the post. Burns had previously worked in the Children's Department of the Tavistock and at various London hospitals. At a later date, and as we saw in chapter 1, he was to take up a Commonwealth Fund Fellowship which was used to travel to the Continent to study child guidance techniques. In any event, the clinic finally opened in April 1932.[32]

In financial and administrative terms the next important step came as Birmingham's Education Committee began to discuss what to do once the voluntary monies had run out. Before this, though, wider discussions had been taking place.

In July 1933 Moodie and Priscilla Norman, in their respective capacities as General Secretary to the CGC and Chair of its Executive Committee, met with Dr Ralph Crowley and Mr Maudslay at the Board of Education. Crowley, who had been involved with child guidance from the outset, was the Board's Senior Medical Officer while Maudslay was its secretary. This meeting followed representations from the Child Guidance Clinic at the West End Hospital for Nervous Diseases that local authorities should be allowed to contribute towards clinic costs. The visitors pointed out that child guidance presently gained Commonwealth Fund financial support but that this would diminish over time. In a rather opaque piece of reasoning Norman also suggested that the 'fact that the work of the Clinics depended on voluntary contributions strengthened the suspicion which still existed in many minds that they were in some way related to "psycho-analysis"'. It was thus desirable that 'some official form of encouragement should be given to their work, and that the State should formally recognise its importance'. Maudslay expressed sympathy while pointing to the country's current financial crisis (ironically, given that Mrs Norman was married to the Governor of the Bank of England). Crowley intervened to suggest that only a small amount of funding would be necessary and his colleague agreed to consider the matter further.[33]

This he duly did, soliciting such opinions as that of Sir George Newman. Maudslay commented that previous refusals to fund child guidance had been due not to any doubts about its value but rather because 'our authority to approve new expenditure on the School Medical Service only covers urgently needed developments' in its main functions. However, given the representations of the Council and of the West End Hospital, Maudslay stated: 'I think we should be justified in modifying our practice. It appears to be generally agreed that the total amount which LEAs are likely to wish to contribute will, for some years at any rate, be quite small'. Newman agreed although in the short term payments continued to be blocked by the Board on the grounds of expenditure constraints.[34] Nonetheless the principle of direct local authority support for child guidance had been established and was duly noted by the Board.[35]

By early 1935 LEAs were allowed to count referral to a child guidance clinic as school attendance and to make contributions to any voluntary clinics to which pupils were referred. These rather abstruse, technical points effectively meant that local authorities could, with the Board's permission, set up their own child guidance clinics and Birmingham took advantage of this situation. Board officials emphasized that 'while the strict embargo [on this form of expenditure] has been raised we are dealing very cautiously with applications and considering each one on its merits'.[36] A Board delegate to a child guidance conference in 1937 stressed that the time had not yet come to 'insist on Local Authorities providing Child Guidance as a public service'. This careful approach was justified on the grounds that of 'all the services, it requires the most skilled personnel and the most delicate of techniques, and would inevitably suffer by methods of mass production'.[37] But the relationship had nonetheless been established. The CMO explained that this was in 'line with the general principles of English educational administration' which involved ascertaining the worth of any new development under voluntary provision and then permitting 'extensions by Local Authorities in suitable cases which are kept under review'.[38]

All the caution, constraints, technicalities and bureaucratic manoeuvrings notwithstanding this was a crucial moment in British child guidance history. Official recognition must be seen not only as important in its own right but as also paving the way for the legislation of the 1940s and thereby local authority predominance in child guidance provision. It was, in addition, a much more generally applicable form of recognition than that accorded to the LCC in the late 1920s. And, too, it can be seen as part of a broader political and public interest in and support for child guidance. It is also important to recall the Commonwealth Fund's long-term strategy. This involved establishing British child guidance while making it clear that financial support would be progressively withdrawn to be replaced by local sources. In fact this was not really to happen until the 1940s and voluntary activity continued to have a part to play, not least through the activities of the CGC and its successor bodies. A new era had nonetheless arrived.

Back in Birmingham this shift was recognized by the Education Committee. In autumn 1934 its Child Guidance Clinic Sub-Committee noted the imminent demise of voluntary funding. The number and type of cases referred, though, suggested an 'urgent need for the continued provision of treatment'. The results achieved implied that the methods employed by the clinic team were on 'sound lines'. Clinic staff consisted of Burns, a psychologist and a PSW. The first two were able to devote three half days per week to child guidance activities (both had other official responsibilities). One consequence of this time limitation was that the clinic's activities tended to focus on only part of the city – the north and north-east – although patients could be referred from outside these districts. The report concluded by urging the clinic's continuance using local authority funding although it was acknowledged that the Board of Education, 'while cognizant of the establishment of the clinic and ... in sympathy with work being carried on therein' had not as yet recognized expenditure on child guidance. The last point notwithstanding, the Committee concurred.[39]

Commentary and data from the late 1930s illustrate the growth and development of clinic's activities. The number of patients referred had risen from 182 in 1932 to around 250 in 1938, that is, by approximately 35 per cent. Of the 250 some 50 per cent of referrals had been initiated by head teachers and medical officers with the rest coming from a variety of sources, including parents. The clinic by 1938 had the voluntary services of two additional psychiatrists, a full-time psychologist and a playroom supervisor. The last was on loan from Margaret Lowenfeld's clinic in London and had had four years of training at the Institute of Child Psychology. The upgrading of the psychologist's post, meanwhile, marked 'a certain change in policy' as it was felt that the 'full observation and study of cases by the Psychologist should include not only testing and remedial coaching, but also observation in the play-room'. The Birmingham system was modelled on Lowenfeld's and hence on the premise that for the child, play was 'his work and his most vital activity through which he learns external reality, develops his personality, and relieves tensions and conflicts'. Patients attended twice-weekly and it was through the observation of play that 'internal evidence' was obtained for diagnosis. This was because the child patient's 'inner life' was revealed 'through the medium of play, since [feelings, desires and imagination] cannot for the most part be expressed in words, especially in the case of younger children'. Play materials were specifically designed for diagnostic purposes so that, for instance, various model figures and model trees, houses and fences could be brought together in a sandpit to create a 'world' of the child's 'fancy'. Play was to be 'as free and spontaneous as possible' and the trained observers should remain 'as unobtrusive and impersonal as possible, not creating emotional relations with the child'.[40]

Play's significance as a diagnostic tool is worth stressing as this was one way in which British child guidance differed from its American counterpart. It could also be used as a form of treatment as we shall see in a specific case from Liverpool in the next chapter. As the training of the Birmingham playroom supervisor suggests, the paediatrician and child psychiatrist Margaret Lowenfeld was a key figure in promoting these ideas. Urwin observes that Lowenfeld was not 'strictly speaking part of the child guidance movement per se although her work later contributed greatly to it' and this sort of tangential relationship characterized Lowenfeld's more general engagement with various strands of psychological and medical research (research being her principle interest).[41] More immediately, Birmingham's utilization of play also gave an opportunity for the psychologist to take on a more clinical role. The latter was, of course, exactly the sort of position psychologists themselves were arguing should be ascribed to their profession.

To return to the spread of clinics, if Birmingham was in the vanguard of child guidance provision outside London, other cities and towns too began to address the issue of maladjusted children. In Manchester a voluntary clinic was founded in 1933 and taken over by the city's education authority in 1937. By the latter date it had another prominent figure in British child guidance, the psychiatrist Mary Burbury, as Medical Director.[42] In 1936 a clinic was opened in Bristol thanks, according to a later official account, to the enthusiasm and commitment of local lay people and in particular Lady Inskip, wife of a leading politician and member of an influential Bristol family. The pre-war years, this report continued, saw 'steady growth' and the participation on a voluntary basis of a number of local psychiatrists.[43] Commenting on this clinic, *Mental Welfare* noted that it had been set up by the LEA and that as such the latter was the third to 'avail itself of the recognition now accorded to Child Guidance Clinics by the Board of Education and their eligibility for Treasury grants'. It was thus 'anticipated that others will follow suit'.[44] Sure enough a year later the same journal announced the opening of a clinic in Sheffield run by a consortium of local authorities. The clinic's advent, it was claimed, had 'aroused an extraordinary amount of interest in the area, which has given great encouragement to its promoters'.[45]

In Liverpool a Child Guidance Council and Clinic was set up in 1929.[46] The clinic started operating in 1930 and in that year dealt with forty-seven referrals. The following year it dealt with 103 patients and by 1939 this had risen to 233. In this report, produced just after the outbreak of the Second World War, particularly detailed data was also given on the source of referrals. Although subject to fluctuations it was generally the case that around 10 per cent of cases came directly from parents. The largest single source was usually schools and education authorities – around one-third in 1939. The report noted, though, the 'marked increase in the number of cases referred by doctors and hospitals'. Again in 1939, this constituted just over one-fifth of referrals. This trend was 'encouraging... as an indication of the close connection between psychology and the field of general medicine'.[47]

Child guidance in Liverpool had some eminent supporters. Council members included Eleanor Rathbone, the social scientist A. M. Carr-Saunders and the city's bishop and archbishop. In the first instance the clinic was financially supported by donations from the Liverpool Council for Social Service and other voluntary bodies. This funding was reasonably generous and allowed for the employment of a social worker, a clerk and a cleaner. Other staff, volunteers from the University and from local hospitals, included three doctors, two paediatricians, an educational psychologist, a speech therapist and a hearing specialist.[48] The relatively healthy level of voluntary donations notwithstanding, in 1934 the Council's Education Committee agreed to donate £100 to the clinic and by the outbreak of war this had increased to £300.[49] The clinic's 1939 annual report recorded further support from the Port Sanitary and Hospitals Committee, the University of Liverpool, the Lancashire Education Committee and nine other local authorities in the region.[50] All this allowed the clinic to remain independent although it was clearly by now highly reliant on public funds. Nonetheless, the geographic area with which it dealt had expanded considerably.

Oxford too had started a clinic and in some respects challenges Birmingham's claim to be the first such institution supported by its local authority – this was certainly suggested by the city's education officer in the mid-1930s.[51] As Board of Education officials likewise noted from 1931, the education authority had 'provided a Clinic in premises lent by the Public Health Department, the expense of

maintenance being estimated at about £150'. However, 'approval of the Authority's proposals was given before the economic crisis of 1931' and the latter 'caused
us to put an embargo for the time being on such developments of the School Medical Service'.[52] This is noteworthy in itself, further evidence of the Board's interest
in child guidance prior to more wide-ranging recognition in the mid-1930s.

The Oxford case was, though, rather complicated. Its so-called 'Educational
Clinic' was ostensibly 'organized on the lines of a Child Guidance Clinic'. But,
notwithstanding that it was led by a retired psychiatrist, it had been set up as
a response to the report of the 1929 Mental Deficiency Committee and from
such accounts as exist appears to have had a very mixed clientele. This ranged
from those who had some form of mental deficiency to cases which appear to
have been much more of the type conventionally dealt with by child guidance
(although, revealingly, some of these were also referred to as 'retarded', suggesting at the very least a particularly acute lack of definitional clarity). It is also
unclear whether local authority funding continued during the financial crisis or
indeed how much was actually incurred.[53] There appears to have been little or no
interaction with the Commonwealth Fund or the CGC. The latter had certainly
recognized the clinic by 1939 and noted that it was now wholly maintained by
its local authority. It was, though, in the category described as: 'Under medical direction but without a fully qualified psychologist and/or psychiatric social
worker'.[54] The central point is that the CGC's approach was that it dealt with
maladjusted, not mentally defective, children. Of course some of the latter inevitably appeared at clinics but they were sent on to the appropriate authorities
rather than dealt with in situ. Perhaps what the Oxford case ultimately illustrates
is that what the CGC thought of as child guidance was not universally understood, adhered to or a matter of agreement.

Definitional problems and the very diversity of provision make it difficult to
be entirely accurate about how many clinics existed by the end of the 1930s. The
Feversham Committee, reporting in 1939, suggested forty-six for Great Britain,
although it is more likely that this actually means England. Different practices
and approaches were acknowledged with some clinics being primarily interested
in the 'dissemination of knowledge among parent-teacher groups or in the education of teachers' while others were 'concerned primarily with the training of
social workers'.[55] In an undated memorandum, probably from early in the war,
the APSW suggested forty-nine clinics for England and Wales of which twenty-
one were wholly or partially maintained by a local authority. Of the total the vast
majority were 'under medical supervision', although by the same token twenty-
one lacked a fully qualified psychologist and/or a psychiatric social worker.[56] As
we shall see in the next section, to this can be added around twelve for Scotland
– hence roughly sixty for Great Britain as a whole.

Whatever the precise figures, three points are clear. First, the number of clinics had risen markedly over the course of the late 1920s and the 1930s. And, as we have seen of individual clinics, the number of children referred had likewise risen sharply. While the source of these referrals was generally from educators, parents too were utilizing child guidance services. Second, the shift had begun from what was essentially a service funded through various forms of voluntary contribution to one in which the state was beginning to play an important role. There was thus a 'mixed economy' of child guidance provision. Third, the child guidance message was increasingly penetrating the broader society through various media and events. As we now turn to examine the situation in Scotland, we will find that while in important respects child guidance there was markedly different from that in England and Wales nonetheless it too conformed to these general trends.

The Peculiarities of the Scots: Catholic Clinics

Although the precise origins of Scottish child guidance were highly contested one early initiative came in 1931 from the Scottish Association for Mental Welfare (SAMW). In a letter circulated to potentially interested parties the Association noted the 'rapid developments which are at present taking place in the field of Education, Psychology and Psychiatry'. Consequently, the SAMW was 'interesting itself in the Child Guidance Movement'. The field was 'not the task of any one profession or section of the Community'. Rather, best results would derive from 'close co-operation between all the agencies concerned with the education of the child, and also with his moral growth'. And so it was 'proposed to launch the Child Guidance Movement in Scotland'.[57] In fact the Association was off the pace here – as we shall see presently, the two Scottish Catholic Clinics were about to be opened.

It was similarly wrong-footed in 1934 when the Scottish Child Guidance Council was launched, largely on MacCalman's initiative. Indicative perhaps of the tensions in child guidance, in Scotland as elsewhere, it was noted that the discussion around the Council's constitution 'took some considerable time'. This was unsurprising given the radically different views held by some of the participants in this process which included the psychologists Boyd and Drever as well as MacCalman.[58] The SAMW's Mental Hygiene Sub-Committee wrote to the new organization pointing out, rather huffily, that 'confusion might arise from duplication of Bodies engaged in this work' and that it had 'already done much propaganda work in this connection and had been recognized by the International Council for Mental Hygiene' as the Scottish body to deal with all mental hygiene matters.[59] Such slights notwithstanding the Mental Hygiene Sub-Committee included, at various points, leading figures in Scottish child guidance, such as Sister Marie Hilda, Drever, Boyd and Henderson. The SAMW merged with the Scottish Child Guidance Council in 1938 to form the Scottish Association for Mental Hygiene.[60] Despite this somewhat farcical start, Scottish child guidance began to take off in the 1930s.

It was, though, notably different from its interwar English counterpart in two, rather contradictory, ways: through the presence of two specifically Catholic institutions and through, outside of these, the dominance of educational psychology. Both Catholic clinics were set up in 1931. In Edinburgh the driving force was Lady Margaret Kerr although, her formidable personality notwithstanding, this clinic was to struggle. The Glasgow institution, set up as an adjunct to the Notre Dame Teacher Training College, was founded by Sister Marie Hilda, a trained psychologist who had started the clinic at the urging of a colleague at Glasgow's other teacher training college.[61] MacCalman was the Notre Dame Clinic's first established Medical Director. In contrast to the Edinburgh Catholic clinic, the one in Glasgow was viewed, not least by supporters of the Commonwealth Fund and CGC approach, as a great success.[62]

Moodie, for example,

> gave an extremely favourable report [to the CGC] on the work that was being undertaken ... and in his conversations with various important persons in the City, he learnt of the excellent impression it was making in both Catholic and non-Catholic circles.

These observations were then forwarded to the Commonwealth Fund.[63] This positive view was shared by a Fund official who visited the clinic early in 1933. Notre Dame seemed, he reported, 'more firmly established' than other clinics he had observed. This was due to the 'remarkable organizing ability of Sister Marie Hilda'. The premises were good and more attractive than in any other provincial clinic and

> the playroom where the children wait for their interviews and where they have play opportunities planned in connection with treatment, is one of the most beautiful Child Guidance Clinic rooms I have seen either in England [*sic*] or in America.[64]

The role of play is again notable here. Notre Dame received a wide variety of visitors, a further means by which the child guidance message was spread. So, for instance, the Scottish branch of the BPS paid a call in March 1934 during which they heard a paper by MacCalman: 'A Comparative Study of Normal and Problem Children, as Revealed by the Rorschach Test'.[65] The clinic's annual report for around the same period recorded over 200 visitors, including social science students at Glasgow University and overseas visitors from as far afield as China and Malaya.[66]

In both Edinburgh and Glasgow the Catholic proponents of child guidance were fortunate in that they gained support from their respective archbishops. In Edinburgh a leaflet designed to inform parents of the clinic's activities stressed that: 'His GRACE THE ARCHBISHOP OF EDINBURGH is glad that Catholic children should have the help of the Clinic' while the annual report for 1934–5 noted that 'His Grace Archbishop MacDonald welcomed the establishment of this unit in his diocese, and Edinburgh was thus the first city in the United Kingdom in which a Catholic Child Guidance Clinic was set up'.[67] Rather cynically, Moodie told Scoville that the archbishop 'gave me the impression he was doing what he could to help the Clinic merely because Lady Margaret Kerr, who organises it, is one of his wealthy and influential parishioners' although as we have seen it was precisely such 'wealthy and influential' individuals whose support the Fund sought.[68]

Over in Glasgow a report on the work of Notre Dame Training College from the early 1930s noted that the new clinic had attracted support not only from the College itself, in the form of premises, but also through a cheque from one Canon O'Brien and another financial donation from the Sister Superior Provincial of Notre Dame.[69] In 1934, meanwhile, Sister Marie Hilda received a letter from the archbishop of Glasgow. The latter noted his initial concerns about the clinic and his request for further information. This had been duly supplied and he now considered it 'beyond any doubt that the treatment given in the Notre Dame Clinic is really effective'. He thus hoped that 'before long there may be many clinics in Scotland such as Notre Dame'. The archbishop could not conceal, he concluded, the 'fact that I am very proud to think that the Sisters of Notre Dame are pioneers in this work'. Most important of all he attached a cheque.[70]

Sustenance, financial and moral, was received from other Catholic bodies. The St Vincent de Paul Society was persuaded to supply holidays for a number of Edinburgh clinic's patients.[71] This organization had backed Notre Dame too, apparently from the outset.[72] Support was forthcoming also from non-Catholic sources. Both clinics received small grants from the main Scottish teachers' union, the Educational Institute of Scotland (EIS). A crucial difference, though, was the level of support Notre Dame received from the civic authorities and from the Commonwealth Fund. Glasgow Corporation took a very positive approach and increased its subsidy in 1937 from £150 to £300.[73] In Edinburgh, by contrast, the only reference to local authority financial support is a passing comment by Kerr which implied a fairly meagre amount.[74] This may account for a throwaway remark by MacCalman that 'in Edinburgh, a cold wind blows on the Roman faith'.[75] The Fund likewise indirectly supported Notre Dame, which was seen as an exemplary institution, while retaining a highly sceptical attitude towards Edinburgh, which was in a constant state of crisis. Notre Dame – various financial scares notwithstanding – was to survive into the welfare state era as an autonomous body and as at 2012 was still in operation in the same premises to which it relocated after the Second World War, albeit now as a 'Centre' rather than a 'Clinic'.

The support given to both clinics by, most notably, the respective archbishops needs to be seen in the wider context. Catholic advocates had not only to contend with the general criticism to which child guidance was subject. They also had to counter scepticism and hostility from other Catholics. The point was repeatedly made that Sister Marie Hilda was a 'pioneer' and that, as one of her successors was to put it, she had to 'fight apathy, indifference and sheer ignorance of the issues at stake – from all quarters. There was indeed considerable opposition – hers was a voice of one crying in the wilderness of prejudice and distrust'.[76] In his review in the Catholic journal the *Tablet* of a book devoted to Notre Dame – M. D. L. Dickson's *Child Guidance* – Burns remarked that the 'subject of Child Guidance is almost entirely ignored by the Catholic body' and when it was acknowledged met with 'that peculiarly suspicious prejudice arising from a little knowledge plus sectarianism'. Burns found it a 'reproach' that no Catholic clinics existed in England and saw Dickson's book as a 'landmark for all Catholics connected with the education and upbringing of children'.[77]

This hostility operated in different ways. Kerr told a correspondent that: 'We have had a great deal of prejudice to overcome amongst the teachers who are still inclined to think that it's casting a slur on their schools to suggest that they might have problem children'.[78] In one instance an Edinburgh PSW reported on a discussion with the head teacher of St Patrick's School, Sister Lucy. The latter had stated that: 'There is the child who has a kink [presumably MD] and the child who is naughty'. The social worker's report continued that Sister Lucy 'cannot believe that a mother would hate a child or a child his parent but supposes it happens in rare cases'.[79] This disinclination to accept the purported insights of the relatively new scientific discipline of psychology was more forcefully expressed in a leading article in the *Tablet*. Describing a child's first communion, the author then remarked on how 'pitiful beside this is the modern cult of "the child" and "its" psychology'. The modern world was making a 'tragedy' of its childhood. Such a modern world 'with its talk of self-expression and the development of "personality"' had 'no real conception of the dignity which God has given to Manhood'. How, then could it have any conception of the 'dignity of Childhood'?[80]

This is a revealing argument not least for the repeated, and pejorative, use of the word 'modern'. Sister Marie Hilda and her colleagues were consciously and explicitly part of a broader movement for Catholic Action which saw itself as taking on the problems thrown up by modernity rather than simply passively disliking, but accepting, them. And one of the tools this struggle would utilize was the 'new psychology'.[81] Child guidance's role in this social mission was frequently stressed. A Catholic teacher in Fife wrote to the Edinburgh Clinic commending its work and his own attempts to publicize it before concluding: 'With every good wish for the success of your labours in this interesting and admirable field of Catholic action'.[82] On a broader front – and almost certainly alluding to contemporary interest in issues such as eugenics, sterilization and birth control – one of the Edinburgh clinic's leading supporters expressed the hope that 'Catholics in general' might take a 'greater interest in the movement for Mental Hygiene which is developing throughout the country and which is in great danger of being entirely swayed by pagan ideas'.[83]

There could be little doubt that for Catholic child guidance supporters this was an explicitly Catholic project. Even Sister Marie Hilda came in for criticism for employing a Protestant psychiatrist, MacCalman.[84] We shortly focus on Sister Marie Hilda and her own and a Glasgow colleague's view of what constituted Catholic child guidance. But this was something which concerned all Scottish Catholic supporters. The Edinburgh clinic's psychiatrist, Dr Mildred Macgown, wrote to the archbishop of St Andrews and Edinburgh in 1934 urging the appointment of a clinic chaplain. While the tools of psychology were undoubtedly useful, Macgown could not help feeling that

> we are missing the main issue. Our Clinic is a Catholic Clinic; we are dealing with Catholic children, and it seems to me that a Catholic child cannot begin to realise too early that in every difficulty or problem he can find the help he needs in his faith, and especially the Sacraments of the Church.

No permanent good could be done, therefore, until 'we apply Catholic remedies to abnormal mental tendencies, and we can only do this with the help of a priest who is interested and in sympathy with the work' and had the time to study cases and attend case conferences.[85]

Either directly as a result of this intervention or for other, associated, reasons, a chaplain was appointed shortly thereafter. As Kerr told a correspondent it had always been the Edinburgh clinic's 'determined policy' that all staff members were practising Catholics. In certain cases, moreover, the Clinic chaplain saw patients and 'he is always present at Case Conferences'. 'The religious element', she commented, was 'always taken into account during investigations' and advice given which 'accords with the moral teaching of the Church'. Everything was hence being done 'to help the patient live a normal Catholic life'.[86]

The issue here was not simply what went on in Catholic clinics themselves. With an increasing number of secular clinics being founded, there was a perceived danger that without either a clear Catholic alternative or at the very least Catholic representation on, especially, local authority clinics, harmful advice might be given. It is thus unsurprising that the records of the Edinburgh clinic contain a cutting from the *Universe* of an article entitled 'US Priest Lectures on Psychology. Stresses Need for Catholic Child Guidance Clinics'. This American guest of the Catholic Psychological Society, after acknowledging Freud while dismissing some of his ideas 'for scientific reasons', noted that 'Catholics are not immune from the various psychical ills which beset mankind'. There were as yet, though, very few Catholic institutions where these could be addressed and in consequence 'Catholic sufferers from mental ailments were, for the most part, forced to seek treatment from non-Catholic organizations, often with very undesirable results'.[87]

What, though, of the frequently embattled pioneer who nonetheless believed that, as she put it herself, God generally wanted what she wanted.[88] Close to the end of her life Sister Marie Hilda wrote a brief work entitled *Child Guidance*. This noted that in the twenty years since its inception her clinic had seen some 2,500 patients. These had come from all sections of society and while it was certainly the case that the majority had been Catholics, nonetheless children from a wide range of religious denominations had attended.[89] But there could be no doubt for Sister Marie Hilda about the principles underpinning the clinic and its approach. It was 'essentially' a Catholic institution with a chaplain appointed by the archbishop of Glasgow. The chaplain's duty was to advise staff on ethical issues 'and to help in the diagnosis and readjustment of the child's behaviour where the cause is due to religious difficulties'. 'Catholicity', the author continued, 'is not a separate department of life, it is an all-pervading influence'.[90] Sister Marie Hilda thus found it appropriate to address theological criticisms of child guidance theory and practice.[91]

To give a sense of Sister Marie Hilda's approach let us take the question of original sin. Opponents of child guidance had argued that the latter discredited the notion of 'perverse conduct as a consequence of original sin' because of the emphasis laid on the child's environment. Sister Marie Hilda agreed that such criticism was partially justified because the clinic did indeed 'tend to lay the chief burden of responsibility on those in authority over the child'. But, she continued,

> is it not just in the ease with which bad example is followed that the effect of original sin is manifested? All Catholics would surely agree that the number of problem children would be infinitely less, if ideal family conditions existed as in the home of St Teresa of Lisieux. Hence, might it not be better to stress more the effects of the Sacrament of Baptism rather than those resulting from original sin?[92]

The theological validity or otherwise of this argument is not the issue here – rather, what is important is that Sister Marie Hilda, one of the leading Catholic proponents of child guidance and of the efficacy of the new psychology, chose to take on critical fellow Catholics in theological debate.

Actual Catholic child guidance practice can be illustrated by a case documented in Dickson's book.[93] This concerned an 8-year-old child of average intelligence from a good Catholic home wherein the child was well cared for and, as Dickson put it, 'brought up carefully'. The child had, though, been caught 'indulging in sex play with other children' and had been brought to the clinic. This type of case was not uncommon in child guidance clinics but at Notre Dame analysis and treatment involved fairly standard psychiatric approaches alongside those which were specifically Catholic. During the latter approach it was noted that the child had realized that he or she (the gender is not specified) had done 'wrong' and had been to Confession. Under the 'wise guidance of the parish priest' the patient was 'making a good adjustment'.

There was, however, a problem with the mother. Her attitude to the incident, as revealed in particular to the PSW, was one of 'almost abnormal horror and repulsion' and through her 'constant expression of intense dislike and shame, was undoing all that was being done to help the patient'. She had a 'misguided view of purity', stressing the negative rather than the positive about sexual intercourse, which she regarded as 'horrible and loathsome'. 'Even her own married life', it was asserted, 'she inclined to view in this light'. Dickson claimed that a non-Catholic social worker might well have told the mother that 'her own attitude to sex was wrong, that there was no need to have any sense of guilt about these matters, that the whole Christian and Catholic attitude was mistaken' much to the detriment of both mother and child. Given the interaction of social workers and patients and their families this explains Dickson's insistence and that of fellow Catholic child guidance supporters that in Catholic clinics PSWs had to be practising Catholics.

In this particular case the mother and social worker engaged in a dialogue with the former coming to see that she 'had failed absolutely to understand and appreciate the dignity and beauty of sex as shown forth in wedlock, how the Church teaches that marriage is a great Sacrament, not a bondage for the avoidance of sin'. In the end the mother began to change her attitude, to her own and her family's benefit. It is worth noting that here again we find instances in child guidance of the focus shifting from the child to one of the parents, specifically the mother, and of the social worker's interventionist role. But the centrality of Catholicism is further made explicit in a comment made by one of the Edinburgh PSWs. Child guidance was, she claimed, 'responsible work' and not least because it dealt 'with the soul'.[94] This was some way from the purportedly non-moralistic and scientific approaches which other child guidance supporters advocated.

In the 1930s Catholic child guidance was a uniquely Scottish phenomenon. Both clinics adhered, at least in principle, to the American/medical model. But they also saw themselves as part of a broader Catholic project which sought both to engage with the problems of modernity while resisting what were perceived as secular practices incompatible with Catholicism. This was most obviously manifested in the use of priests although the insistence that at the very least PSWs should be Catholic was also important. Such commitment to a particular set of religious beliefs notwithstanding, Notre Dame, if not the Edinburgh clinic, was looked upon favourably by the Commonwealth Fund which sought to use it as a bridgehead into wider Catholic circles. Events were, though, to overtake this strategy and although a sister clinic to that in Glasgow was founded in Liverpool in the early 1940s British child guidance was, through its appropriation by the state, largely to follow a different path. The Scottish Catholic clinics, and especially Notre Dame, were nonetheless an important development in their own right as well as illustrating an underexplored part of modern British welfare history, the provision of social services by religious bodies. But what of the non-Catholic clinics in Scotland?

The Peculiarities of the Scots: Psychology

As seen in the previous chapter there can be little doubt that in the interwar period psychology as a discipline and profession was in a relatively weak position in English child guidance. The situation in Scotland, though, was notably different. This was remarked upon at the time by MacCalman. He generously observed that, the medical model notwithstanding, the 'earliest clinics were organized and directed by lay psychologists – Prof. Drever's clinic in Edinburgh and Dr Boyd's clinic in Glasgow'. This was partly due, he suggested less charitably, to the 'traditional over emphasis on education in Scotland' as well as to the 'dearth of psychiatrists trained in child guidance, the unwillingness of local authorities to embark on the necessary expenditure, and the willingness of university departments of psychology and education to do this work voluntarily'.[95] The different trajectory of Scottish child guidance was further underpinned by the country's separate systems of education and teacher training. As we shall see in chapter 6, the Scottish version of child guidance came to be regarded as the way forward in the 1940s and was thus an important factor in the shift away from psychiatry to psychology.[96]

For the most part Scottish child guidance clinics in the interwar era followed the pattern suggested by MacCalman and in particular through their focus on educational psychology rather than psychiatry. Sir Alexander Macgregor, recalling his time as Glasgow's MOH, remarked that in the 1930s he had watched Notre Dame's work with 'growing admiration'. Nonetheless when he and his counterpart in the Education Department decided to create a local authority child guidance service in 1937 it was to be 'conducted by trained teacher psychologists [afterwards officially called educational psychologists]'. A special course in child guidance for teachers had been available at Jordanhill Teacher Training College since 1934 and while psychiatric help was available to the clinic it is clear from Macgregor's account that this was to be very much a last resort, with educational psychology taking the lead.[97]

In fact, and to reinforce the point, the person appointed to lead this new municipal service was the protégé of Boyd alluded to in the previous chapter, Catherine McCallum. A later account suggests that the decision to set up this service arose from a delegation consisting of representatives from the Scottish Child Guidance Council, Notre Dame and Boyd's clinic to Glasgow Corporation, their argument being that a city of Glasgow's size should not have to rely in what was essentially voluntary provision. The Corporation clinic saw nearly 250 cases in its first year, almost all of whom had been referred by teachers, and was administered on behalf of the Education Committee by the educational psychologist. The referrals were predominantly on account of 'unmanageable behaviour, aggression, and temper tantrums' with, rather unusually, relatively few cases of bed-wetting. A further municipal clinic was opened in June 1939.[98]

In an important symposium held in the early 1950s on the respective roles of psychiatry and psychology in child guidance, McCallum conceded that Scottish child guidance had been 'characterised more by diversity than uniformity', although in fact this was true of child guidance more generally. Nonetheless, it 'began in the universities' – here she was referring to the work of Boyd and Drever – before being taken up by teacher training colleges. Members of the teaching profession had been the 'outstanding personalities in the movement' and had persuaded local authorities to support child guidance in advance of statutory permission. And so, on a 'purely factual basis' Scottish child guidance had long 'been established ... as an educational service' and this explained the 'very favourable position' enjoyed by psychologists. Such psychologists were, she explained, non-medical individuals with an honours degree in psychology and almost all had trained as teachers.[99]

The points made by McCallum are illustrated by the cases of Edinburgh and Dundee. The capital's local authority certainly debated the setting up of its own child guidance clinic in the 1930s and sent representatives to bodies such as the Scottish Child Guidance Council. It also utilized Drever's University-based clinic, especially for stammerers.[100] Nonetheless, an Edinburgh Corporation publication from the mid-1930s noted that while there were two clinics in the city – almost certainly the struggling Catholic clinic and Drever's psychological clinic – both were run on a voluntary basis and no indication was given that the Corporation itself planned to enter the field.[101] Indeed, although by 1939 there were now three clinics, it remained the case that none were run by the local authority.[102]

In Dundee the body responsible for teacher training in the area had set up a 'Psychological Clinic' in 1932 at the behest of the local branch of the SAMW. It was noted a year later that while only a small number of cases had been dealt with, and while this work had been useful and remedial work could be successfully carried out within the confines of the teacher training college, nonetheless such an arrangement could 'never adequately meet the needs of a city the size of Dundee'.[103] Consequently the city council was approached for help and in due course agreed to a financial subsidy for the clinic.[104] Further subsidies were duly acquired, including from the CGC, to aid with the employment of a PSW.[105] So this clinic, like many others in Scotland and elsewhere, was underwritten by a combination of voluntary labour from the teacher training college, charitable subsidies and local authority grants.

How did it operate? It is important to note that it would not have received CGC support had there not been at least some psychiatric input. And as the Dundee MOH noted in the mid-1930s on the formalizing of the clinic's status and its ongoing location in the teacher training college, while child guidance was 'essentially an educational movement' nonetheless 'it undoubtedly has a medical implication'.[106] But it was the first half of this formulation which was, ultimately, the most important. This was for two reasons, the first pragmatic, the second more fundamental. First, when the clinic was being set up it was beyond the 'bounds of practical politics' that either a psychiatrist or a PSW could be appointed. In due course, emphasis was duly and successfully placed on acquiring the latter. Second, in any event the 'great majority' of cases were psychological or educational rather than psychiatric. More than this, while the need for a clinic had certainly been recognized,

> we have never lost sight of two principles which were formulated early in our discussions, namely, that the Clinic should be an integral part of the education system of the city, and that it should be run in close association with the Training College.[107]

So by the late 1930s the clinic was described as 'fully equipped and adequately staffed' since it employed a full-time psychologist and a full-time PSW. All this might be seen as a very limited victory for the CGC in terms of its investment but, once again, it can also be seen as a further assertion of the dominance in Scotland of psychology. And while the support of those psychiatrists who gave some input was acknowledged – and on occasions patients were referred to Mac-Calman in Aberdeen – it was also noted that the clinic's work was 'providing an invaluable adjunct to the psychological instruction in the Training College'.[108] In short this was a clinic wherein psychiatry was not entirely absent and teamwork certainly took place. Nor is there any evidence of the more or less openly hostile attitude to psychiatry which can be found in the work of, in particular, Boyd. But it was also a clinic closely associated with educational training and run by a psychologist – a very different picture from that which predominated in England. Hence our notion of a Scottish challenge to the American model, a challenge based on the claims of psychology at the expense of those of psychiatry.

This approach was officially approved of, unsurprisingly given the influence of the educational establishment, and not least individuals such as Boyd, on official policy.[109] In 1938 a Scottish Education Department (SED) report noted that child guidance had first been undertaken in Scotland in 1925 at Glasgow University – that is, at Boyd's clinic and thus before the intervention of the Commonwealth Fund or the setting up of the CGC. There were now eleven Scottish clinics, one of which was directly run by a local authority, Glasgow. The rest were organized on a voluntary basis with some receiving grants from Education Authorities or bodies such as the National Committee for the Training of Teachers. Three were attached, 'very fittingly', to teacher training establishments and in 1935/6 Boyd's clinic had, in conjunction with the Provincial Committee for the Training of Teachers, set up a course for in-service teachers attended by sixty-two members of the profession. The value of such clinics' services, the passage concluded, was being increasingly recognized by the 'various bodies and social agencies concerned with the same problems, as well as from teachers and parents, who to-day readily seek advice at the Clinics on the difficulties affecting the individual child'.[110] What is striking here is the absence of any mention of psychiatry, PSWs, the Scottish CGC or the Commonwealth Fund. In line with the broader trend to greater local authority support, by the early 1940s the Scottish Association for Mental Hygiene recognized thirteen Scottish clinics, including three in Edinburgh and four in Glasgow. In Scotland as a whole, seven of the thirteen clinics were now wholly or partially maintained by local authorities.[111]

Conclusion

Although coverage was by no means uniform or complete, nonetheless by the late 1930s child guidance had spread from the confines of London to other areas of Britain. Of course, this statement has to be qualified in the light of what we have seen as the (retrospective) claims of certain Scottish psychological clinics to have led the way in child guidance provision. This in turn highlights not only diversity within Britain but also that this was a contested domain, especially between those who proposed the psychiatrically based American, or medical, model and those who, particularly in Scotland, saw child maladjustment as a behavioural rather than a medical issue and thereby the provenance of psychology. Scotland provided another form of exceptionalism in the shape of its Catholic clinics which, although attuned to modern developments in psychological medicine, nonetheless saw the spiritual dimension as, ultimately, the most important. Less contentiously, perhaps, child guidance had also spread through the commitment of its practitioners and supporters to publishing for and talking to a broad audience, from fellow professionals to the general public. We now move on to examine those whom child guidance was set up to help, its child patients.

4 NORMALCY, HAPPINESS AND CHILD GUIDANCE IN PRACTICE[1]

Introduction

In the last chapter we examined child guidance provision's expansion from its initial location in London, its further recognition by the Board of Education and its spread by way of various media and events and through the activities of supporters and practitioners. We now turn to those at whom child guidance was aimed, the normal child suffering some form of maladjustment, the symptoms of which were various behaviours deemed in some way unacceptable. We thus analyse in more detail what is meant by the concept of 'normalcy' and the significance or otherwise of 'happiness' to a child's mental well-being. Using selected case studies we engage with the diagnosis and treatment accorded to a child patient and its family when referred to a clinic. As will become apparent, child guidance's focus quickly shifted to parents and particularly the mother. All these concerns and activities were allegedly in pursuit of better mental hygiene for children, their families and the broader society.

In Search of the Normal Child

Notwithstanding their different functions and aspirations, the three child guidance professions were anxious to promote their own, and child guidance's, scientific credentials. A further unifying feature was their concern with the normal child – that is the child who at some point in his or her emotional and psychological development might become maladjusted but who, through the intervention of the child guidance team, could be returned to normalcy. Achieving normalcy, though, was not unproblematic. For one thing, there was the nature of the interwar period itself. It was a 'commonplace', claimed the Feversham Committee, that 'the times in which we are living are not normal'. All social classes were experiencing 'anxiety, uncertainty and strain in varying degrees' induced by the 'increasing speed of life made possible by scientific progress'. Hence what would 'otherwise be latent maladjustment of an unimportant kind is liable to become serious mental disorder'.[2] A group of London Clinic supporters wrote to *The Times* in 1937 that there was a 'grave menace of mental disorder among children' and that even allowing for the present economic crisis, the 'the need of the sick in mind requiring help and adjustment' was as great as that of the physically ill.[3] These comments echo those encountered previously regarding the psychological problems engendered by modernity.

There were also problems of definition and measurement. Moodie told a professional audience in 1929 that great advances had been made in child psychology through methods such as intelligence testing. Attempts to devise equivalent tests for 'emotional or temperamental evaluation' had, though, so far been unsuccessful.[4] A few years later Burns, reviewing the results of the Birmingham clinic's work, rather defensively remarked that 'facts and estimates' were difficult to translate into hard data since 'there can be no fixed standard'.[5] In his pre-war survey of child guidance, meanwhile, MacCalman argued that treatment continued to be hampered because 'our understanding of what is normal in emotional development is incomplete and meagre'.[6]

Rather more positively, Moodie also noted that all 'normal children are difficult at times' and the 'average parent' was perfectly capable of dealing with such disturbances.[7] Nonetheless, and again to complicate matters, there were significant individual variations within the child population as a whole and hence 'treatment which would have no serious effect upon one child may profoundly influence another'. It was thus difficult to give precise advice in any particular case without knowing the full circumstances of the situation.[8] In the latter part of the war Dr Frank Bodman of the Bristol Child Guidance Clinic remarked that while it was possible to make a fairly accurate assessment of a child's intellectual capacity 'the measurement of emotional development cannot as yet be so mathematically standardised'. Study of the child's behaviour would, Bodman felt, nonetheless allow for 'some rough conclusion about his progress'. But he too acknowledged that each child had to be individually treated. So some 'temperaments take life easily, some make heavy weather of normal problems. Some have an active imagination, others a dull intelligence'. In a rather disingenuous shift of focus, although as we shall see below one which was by this point now well-established, it was thus the parents' responsibility to recognize these traits, and give each child the most favourable circumstances, the optimum atmosphere for its development.[9]

As is evident from the comments of Moodie and Bodman in particular, child guidance was attuned to the concept of the psychology of individual differences as advanced by, notably, Burt. As the psychologist from the Edinburgh Child Guidance Clinic told an official enquiry into delinquency in 1945, she was strongly of the opinion that 'there is no clear distinction between the delinquent and the non-delinquent ... there is no sharp line of cleavage'. Rather, it was always a matter of degree 'and whether it be intellectual, emotional, or a difference of character, it is a problem of individual differences, and a delinquent is not a type apart'.[10] And of course age too had to be taken into account, with different behaviours 'normal' at some ages but not others. MacCalman observed that children passed through 'various stages of emotional growth' and hence that 'certain forms of behaviour are characteristic of these periods'. So, for example, it was 'quite normal for babies to suck their thumbs, for three year olds to have temper tantrums, and for the adolescent to be moody'. But, by contrast, behaviour such as 'moody shyness in a five year old' was 'at least unusual and may be a symptom of neurosis'. To further complicate matters, at times of 'great emotional stress' regression was to be expected.[11]

In short, normalcy and abnormalcy, adjustment and maladjustment were not absolutes. Rather, they could be placed on a spectrum just like intellectual endowment or body weight. The child's stage of emotional and psychological development also had to be taken into account alongside an acknowledgement of his or her own individual characteristics. Such a view added to, rather than diminished, the precariousness of child mental health. If the boundaries between the normal and the abnormal were not clearly defined, if normalcy was constantly under threat and if different children had different responses to the same treatment, then all the more need for vigilance and the surveillance of the child population and children's parents. As Armstrong puts it, 'multiple axes' came to be used to locate the child and its characteristics and as such each individual was categorized not primarily as an autonomous entity but in relation to others – hence the bringing of 'all the significant characteristics of childhood under the monitoring eye of medicine'.[12]

And despite the agonizing about a lack of means to measure emotional development, child guidance practitioners, whether or not they themselves were fully convinced of the categories they employed, nonetheless sought to identify and classify symptoms, underlying aetiologies and maladjustment itself. In the early 1930s a PSW wrote that 'abnormal behaviour', the outward manifestation of maladjustment, might include

> truancy, thieving, moodiness, violent temper, outbursts, backwardness with average intelligence, persistent fantasy formation, unmanageableness, and anything that would suggest the child is not adapting himself in a satisfactory way to his environment; also children suffering from nervous instability showing by stammering and speech defects.[13]

But of course symptoms were not causes. Moodie's colleague, the PSW Pauline Shapiro, noted that some children 'failed to fit into their surroundings' and that their maladjustment was seen in a range of behavioural symptoms. But to call such children incorrigible, nervy, highly strung or backward was to 'describe the symptoms but to explain nothing'.[14] The disjuncture between symptoms and causes and hence the need to find the latter rather than simply treating the former is brought out in a report from Notre Dame. This recorded that the single largest proportion of cases – over half those currently open – had been referred for behaviour disorder such as stealing, temper tantrums and bullying. However, on clinical investigation they had to be reclassified, with the 'real trouble' arising from 'disorders of the personality or in some physical defect'. On reclassification, only 2 per cent of open cases were found to be attributable to 'behaviour disorder'. What had been revealed was that over half the cases were in fact due to disorders of the personality, defined as 'disorders of mood – lability, depression, anxiety, hypochondriasis, or apathy – feelings of inferiority, rejection, or insecurity, and the shy, shut-in, seclusive, brooding or dreamy personality'. Only 2 per cent were found on diagnosis to be psychotic.[15]

Other clinics undertook similar exercises. At Birmingham an analysis was carried out in the mid-1930s, arising from LEA concerns about juvenile delinquency, of 100 children referred to the clinic for stealing. This behaviour and its causes were subdivided into two groups. The first, consisting of 'social, economic, and other environmental conditions', Burns considered 'secondary causes'. The primary, more fundamental, causes were attributable to 'intelligence, personality, and intimate family relationships'. It was therefore possible to distinguish between 'opportunistic' and 'emotional' miscreants. The former were influenced more by secondary causes while investigation into the latter showed that their behaviour should be seen 'primarily as symptoms of emotional maladjustment'. The less such children needed to steal the more likely was this to be the case. These patients had to be treated by 'psychological methods' since such behaviour was 'more deeply engrained, more compulsive, than in the general run of casual delinquency' and as such was a symptom of 'a disorder of the whole personality'.[16]

As will be evident, some of the categories and language employed in interwar child guidance lacked a high degree of clinical precision – indeed was closer to normative judgement about what constituted acceptable behaviour than it was to scientific analysis. But it is worth focusing on the notion of the 'shy, shut-in, seclusive, brooding or dreamy personality' referred to in the Notre Dame report. Shyness was seen as a serious problem by child guidance practitioners. Emanuel Miller suggested in *Child Life* that among the '[m]ajor disorders ... arising from a variety of causes' was 'shyness' (in the same piece he also suggested that '[e]xcessive goodness' in a child was also suspect and arose from 'fear of normal instincts').[17] A flyer seeking financial support for the London Clinic claimed that

> Learning to Drive is child's play, compared with – Learning to Live! ... Learning to Live is harder – if courage fails, fears, anxiety, shyness and failure take its place: a crash may mean stealing, violence, rudeness or truancy, and a breakdown is tragic.[18]

This concern with shyness persisted into the post-war era. In Henderson and Gillespie's standard text the chapter on childhood notes among the disorders of personality timidity, sensitiveness, shyness and lack of sociability.[19] In *Mother and Child*, meanwhile, the psychiatrist Helen Gillespie reported that as well as running her child guidance clinic she was seeing pre-school children at a maternity and child welfare centre, as problems such as 'fears, timidity, shyness' could already be found in this age-group.[20]

Why was such an opaque characteristic such as 'shyness' – which can surely exist only, for the most part, in the eye of the beholder – deemed so problematic? It was an issue in America too. Sol Cohen comments that here the quiet, timid, shy or so-called 'good' child was a more serious concern than the 'aggressive child, the child who overtly misbehaved' because the former's problems were potentially more serious and more easily overlooked.[21] Christopher Lane, examining the 'transformation of shyness into a disease', focuses especially on the latter part of the twentieth century. But he also traces the origins of this transformation to psychiatric thought from the last decades of the nineteenth century onwards. The title of his book, *Shyness: How Normal Behaviour Became a Sickness*, sums up the trajectory of his argument with one outcome being, as he puts it, 'a vast, perhaps unrecoverable, loss of emotional range, an impoverishment of human experience'.[22]

Cohen and Lane's arguments help illuminate and contextualize the British experience. And while the medicalization of child shyness has not gone nearly so far in Britain as in the US, Lane's analysis partially qualifies the otherwise useful point made by Hayes. She argues that in the latter part of the twentieth century and into the twenty-first, it is the hyperactive child who is seen as particularly problematic, so that the maladjusted child has gone from being the passive 'rabbit' to the overactive 'rebel'.[23] Whatever the timing and nuances of these developments, concerns over shyness show that certain behaviours deemed acceptable in one historical era may be less so in another. This in turn reinforces the idea that we should question, historically and sociologically, the clinical validity of certain diagnoses and categories. So, and returning to the issue of normalcy and adjustment, we should endorse Turmel's comment that the 'child was recognized as normal when it was classified as such'.[24] And we might also recall Armstrong's observations on the 'problematisation of the normal' and how children were the first target of a shift towards surveying apparently health populations.

More broadly, psychiatrists were confronting a series of problems noted by commentators such as Rose and Rosenberg. Rose observes that 'our own notions of normality and mental disorder are inescapably historically and culturally specific', the logic of which is that the same must have been true in the past. So not only was normalcy part of a spectrum, it was part of a spectrum where the already ill-defined borders between normalcy and abnormalcy shifted over time.[25] Rosenberg, discussing the problems inherent in defining disease, argues that 'behavioural and emotional ailments constitute a particularly sensitive and contingent subset of problems'. Since its emergence as a specialism in the nineteenth century 'psychiatry has been a definer of boundaries, a delineator and designated manager of the normal and the abnormal, and thus unavoidably a key participant in this never-ending debate'. Simultaneously, though, it has 'suffered from a recurrent status anxiety' and been 'chronically' sensitive to its inability to call upon a repertoire of tightly bounded, seemingly objective, and generally agreed-upon diagnostic categories based firmly on biopathological mechanisms'. Hence psychiatry remained the 'legatee of the emotional, the behavioural, and the imperfectly understood'. On the issue of historical specificity Rosenberg suggests that 'behavioral and emotional symptoms are presumed to reflect an underlying mechanism' and are hence in practice 'time- and place-specific vocabularies of disease entities' used for both 'conceptualizing and managing behaviour and feelings'.[26] So, as he puts it in a separate piece, there is an 'endemic boundary conflict' with respect to defining and treating 'ailments whose manifestations are primarily or exclusively behavioral or emotional', ailments potentially ranging from 'what might be called normally distributed variants through what might seem to be incapacitating pathologies'. But, at least as far as the boundaries are concerned, 'where does one draw the line?'[27]

Such analyses allow considerable insight into British child guidance thinking and practice. Indeed some practitioners acknowledged, as we have seen, the difficulty in 'drawing the line' while nonetheless actively doing so themselves. So for child guidance, normalcy was defined by what it was not – a group of historically and socially contingent 'unacceptable' behaviours, the precise contents and acceptability of which might vary over time and between individuals and individual circumstances. There was, furthermore, no sharp boundary between the adjusted and the maladjusted, the normal and the abnormal. And as we shall see there were to be problems in measuring outcomes, thus further muddying the waters.

Are Normal Children Happy?

But first we turn to the issue of happiness which Peter Stearns points to as emerging, in the first decades of the twentieth century, as an aim of childrearing and ideally a condition of childhood itself.[28] Stearns draws his evidence from America, but can such aspirations be found in British child guidance? We have already come across the idea that unhappiness was problematic and symptomatic of deeper-rooted problems. A further instance comes in the remarks of a psychologist from the London Clinic to an education conference in the early 1930s. The unhappy child, she observed, 'is no more competent to profit by school instruction than the child who is physically ill'. To compound the problem a 'child is by no means always able to formulate in words the fact that he is unhappy'. The inevitable result would be either aggressive or infantile behaviour.[29] Burns observed that failure to address the causes of maladjustment, and thereby allowing the child to go on 'being thoroughly unhappy', solved nothing. And as anyone dealing with 'adult neurotics' knew, their childhood was often 'one long tale of unhappiness or mismanagement at home' which could have been prevented by using child guidance services.[30] Moodie likewise told an education conference that there were four types of unstable child: the overactive; the 'shy, quiet' child who 'avoids company, is unpopular, worries, takes things to heart' and who is thus 'internal' rather than 'external'; the child displaying nervous symptoms such as bed-wetting or temper tantrums; and the delinquent. Despite outward differences all four had in common being 'usually tense and highly strung' and this was underpinned by a fundamental anxiety and tension – in short, they were unhappy. Such children usually had, furthermore, 'a high intelligence. The dull child is not usually so anxious or nervous'.[31]

The last point illustrates a more general concern with the particular problems of very intelligent children. As MacCalman put it, clever children 'have just as many problems as the dull and backward, though they may be of a different kind'.[32] To take a specific case embracing both high intelligence and unhappiness, a 9-year-old girl was sent to the Liverpool Clinic in the late 1930s for incontinence and difficult behaviour at school. No physical cause had been identified and psychological testing revealed her to be of 'superior ability'. Psychiatric investigation, though, found the patient 'unhappy and aggrieved, feeling the need for more affection and satisfaction in her daily life'. Treatment had devolved to the PSW, who was working with the mother to help her understand her child's difficulties while the patient herself was attending a weekly play group. All this had resulted in her problems being cleared up.[33]

It might be argued that what is being suggested here are strategies for the avoidance or curing of 'unhappiness' rather than the active promotion of 'happiness' in the manner suggested by Stearns. But in the interwar period it is possible to find examples of child guidance practitioners actively advancing the notion of the 'happy child'. MacCalman addressed 'familiar problems' of childrearing, with especial emphasis on the early years. Such problems could be resolved or avoided, he suggested, through '[l]ove, thought, gentleness, and serenity and a real desire to enter into the life of the child on the part of the parents and to see the child's point of view'. This was, he concluded, 'the basis for an unhampered, sound and happy personality in the child, and for a quiet triumph over the early problems of babyhood'.[34]

The distinction between preventing unhappiness and promoting happiness is to some degree a false one. Nonetheless, the tone and language of much interwar British child guidance discourse leans slightly towards the former rather than the latter. However, we shall see in chapter 5 that, in analyses of wartime evacuation, it was thought that children who were happy in their own homes adapted best to removal from them, while in chapter 6 we find the centrality of children and the family to post-war reconstruction further emphasizing the need for children's mental well-being and, indeed, happiness. Moreover, a further focusing on the centrality of the child–parent relationship and of the experience of the child's earliest years contributed to this refinement of approach. These were pre-figured in the MacCalman extract cited on p. 1 and were to find particular expression in Bowlby's research and publications.

Among Bowlby's most famous works was *Child Care and the Growth of Love*, published in 1953 and hugely influential on British post-war children rearing. But while this was in the first instance based on his report for the World Health Organization, Bowlby was building on long experience, as his opening statement made clear: 'Among the most significant developments of psychiatry during the past quarter of a century' – that is from around the beginnings of British child guidance – 'has been the steady growth of evidence that the quality of parental care' received by a child in the early years was of 'vital importance for his future mental health'. This had led to a consensus among 'child guidance workers in Europe and America' that the infant and young child should 'experience a warm, intimate, and continuous relationship with his mother ... in which both find satisfaction and enjoyment'.[35] So the normal, adjusted child gradually came to be seen also as the happy child, content and solid in its relationships and especially that with its mother.

At the Clinic

So in the event of interwar children being seen as requiring treatment at a child guidance clinic, how would they get there in the first place, how would they be dealt with and by whom, what treatment would be prescribed and with what results? It is important to stress that detailed records, and particularly case notes, have survived in only a relatively small number of instances and that, as was acknowledged at the time, there were variations in practice between clinics. There were also problems of definition and classification which further complicated matters. And of course what is missing altogether is any real sense of the child patient's experience, at least in his or her own voice. Children's feelings, attitudes and behaviours are seen through the prism of the professionals whom they encountered and the latter's clinical preconceptions and, not infrequently, value judgements. What follows, then, can only give an incomplete and partial picture. Nonetheless, the archival and published materials examined are revealing about child guidance practice as it expanded in the 1930s.

Referrals to child guidance clinics came, as we have seen, from a variety of sources. Those by doctors and educationalists were extremely important but by no means the only path by which a child might end up at a clinic. To flesh this out further, and to get a sense of the child patients' intellectual and other characteristics, we focus initially on two Scottish clinics. In the four years up to November

1940 the relatively small Dundee clinic received 339 cases of which about 60 per cent had been sent by a School Medical Officer or the schools themselves. Of the rest the Dundee Royal Infirmary, the children's parents and the juvenile court each contributed around 10 per cent with the remainder being referred by social workers, GPs, speech therapists and other local hospitals.[36] Of course in Scotland, given the dominance of educational psychology and its part in teacher training the high rate of referral by schools and the SMO was to be expected, but it was a pattern not uncommon in the rest of Britain.

A rather different picture, though, emerged at Notre Dame in the late 1930s, at least regarding referrals. Just under 200 new cases had been seen that year. Around 20 per cent had been referred by teachers but the largest single category, around 25 per cent, had been brought by the child's parents. In fact the situation was complicated by a further 12 per cent being sent by a group simply identified as 'physicians', some of whom may have been associated with the School Medical Service. Nonetheless the high proportion of parental referrals is notable, possibly a consequence of Notre Dame's religious orientation but perhaps also an indicator of a more general penetration of the child guidance message. The same report also gives an insight into gender and age. The boy/girl ratio was around 6:4. Age ranged from 18 months to 18 years with around 12 per cent being under school age and around 13 per cent over the school leaving age. The vast majority were thus, as might be expected, schoolchildren although the proportions of younger and older children were not insignificant. The report also gave IQ distribution with 22 per cent above average, 45 per cent average, 22 per cent dull and backward and 11 per cent mentally defective. From the staff's point of view, the PSW had undertaken over 1,200 interviews – in the clinic, at the home, at the school and with other agencies. The psychiatrist had conducted some 1,500 interviews and examinations. It was the psychological interventions which stood out, though, at over 3,000, the bulk of which – nearly 90 per cent – involved 'treatment' consisting of activities such as 'coaching' or running play therapy.[37] This heavy psychological involvement is in part due to the clinic being part of Notre Dame's teacher training function. But it can also be attributed to the significance of play therapy in British child guidance, psychologists' claims to this territory and their associated desire for an explicitly clinical role.

It is important to reiterate the difficulty of generalizing across different clinics. But some general features begin to emerge. An early report from the London Clinic remarked that its patients' IQ distribution was close to that of the general child population.[38] The distribution at Notre Dame can be seen in the same light, a further reminder that child guidance sought to deal with the essentially normal child. Another point which arises from the Notre Dame report is the resource-intensive nature of child guidance, again an issue more broadly recognized. The Liverpool clinic's psychiatrist remarked that if the only benefit of that institution's services was the results achieved in individual cases then it was doubtful whether these were worth the time, money and effort. But justification could be found in child guidance's aim of 'the betterment of the mental health and the behaviour standards of the community as a whole'.[39] The Feversham Committee saw child guidance's resource-intensive nature as a defining characteristic and one which differentiated it from 'older methods which influenced the child by authority or precept' – a further instance of child guidance's purported shift from a moral to a scientific approach. It was thus self-evident that such 'detailed and painstaking study and treatment is costly and time-consuming'.[40]

And, as at Notre Dame, boys generally outnumbered girls, almost certainly a consequence of gendered expectations and the acceptability or otherwise of the sort of activities engaged in by young males. In 1932 the London Clinic saw 276 boys and 200 girls while the East London Clinic took in 129 boys and 48 girls.[41] The small Edinburgh Catholic Clinic took on, in 1933, twenty-one boys and fifteen girls. And to reinforce the point about how resource-intensive child guidance was, these 36 new referrals, combined with the existing 20 cases, engendered 359 social work visits and 187 psychiatric interviews.[42] To generalize broadly, the typical child guidance clinic patient was of between 5 and 14 years of age, had been sent there by the education system, was of average intelligence and was more likely to be a boy than a girl. And while some cases might be disposed of fairly quickly, others had considerable professional resources devoted to them.

But what of the children themselves? We now examine a number of case studies derived from a variety of sources. As we have seen, popular journals such as *Mother and Child* had an overtly didactic purpose and child guidance professionals would use particular cases to illustrate their message. These professionals also wrote for fellow professionals and again case studies were used to back up their scientific argument. And some actual case records can be found in certain archives. To repeat an earlier point – what we are clearly not hearing here are the voices of the children themselves. Rather, we hear of these child patients through the medium of those professionals with whom they came into contact. The aim is not, therefore, to describe the experience of a child at an interwar clinic from that child's perspective, nor is it to claim that the following case studies are 'representative' of the total child patient population. It is also recognized that it was in the interest of the professionals involved, at least when entering the public domain, to validate their own approaches and practices. Rather, the aim is to show how such children were viewed, diagnosed and treated and to deduce what this tells us about child guidance and its ambitions.

M. D. L. Dickson, author of the substantial work on Notre Dame encountered in the last chapter and husband of its PSW, devoted a long passage to 'The Case of Dick'.[43] Dick was a 15-year-old boy performing badly at his boarding school, including cheating in some subjects. He is, though, introduced to us as somebody who is, superficially at least, normal: 'he is quite reasonably good-looking' and has a 'definite charm of manner ... To meet him casually you would not think there was much wrong'. Testing reveals a high IQ, 135. Dick has 'few or no friends' and there was 'abundant suspicion, though no actual proof of sexual malpractices'. What had brought him to the clinic's attention, by way of his school, was a 'series of morbid essays' in which he had exhibited self-disgust. The family circumstances show his father to be 'a highly sensitive man, slightly sentimental perhaps, extremely devoted to his wife, very fond of his son by whom he is utterly perplexed'. The mother, meanwhile, 'seems to be somewhat hard, undemonstrative'. She is nonetheless devoted to her husband while being the household's 'dominant personality'. Another child, John, had died.

At his first meeting with the psychiatrist Dick breaks into hysterical crying. Further meetings ensue, stretching over around two years and the 'picture gradually gets filled in from a series of clues: dreams, old memories, perhaps some of them phantasies, but even if they are they represent the child's feelings at the time'. So it transpires that Dick has always felt that his mother had preferred his now-dead sibling. For this and other reasons he has thus, the psychiatrist suggests to him, been looking to assuage his guilt over John's death and to find a mother substitute by way of a wet nurse and a German maid with whom, Dick blushingly claims, he had 'a romantic episode' when eleven. So, in the interview which marks Dick's breakthrough in terms of understanding and thus a key stage in his adjustment and attainment of normalcy, the psychiatrist claims that his patient is coming to realize the origins of his unhappiness. These lay in part in his unconscious self's struggle to reach maturity and which nearly resulted in 'in killing your power to feel'. Dick's self-realization involves accepting that he is not to blame for his predicament. He then asks who is, and the psychiatrist suggests that while nobody can be 'blamed' nonetheless his parents, while doing their best, had unwittingly made a couple of bad mistakes: 'Net result you have all had to suffer very badly'.

In a subsequent meeting with Dick's headmaster both he and the psychiatrist noted the patient's improvement and his impending university career at 'Oxbridge', the latter unthinkable at the time of the first clinical encounter. Both are agreed that Dick's parents were to blame for his unhappiness, but the psychiatrist explains that the blame 'is really a factual not a moral one' – an interesting, if somewhat implausible, distinction. Essentially, his mother had rejected him during infancy and over-compensated when his brother died, so throwing Dick's emotional world into chaos. The mother was still incapable of expressing her feelings which she 'covers ... in armour plating lest she or anyone else' should see them. In the psychiatrist's view Dick's acquired self-knowledge will help him recover but his parents, filled with guilt and afraid of their own feelings, will continue to suffer.

A general commentary on the case studies is given below but at this stage it is worth making some particular observations about Dick's case. First, he is middle class and highly intelligent, indicators that economic comfort and intellectual ability are of themselves no antidote to maladjustment. Second, by the account which we are given, little is made of the implied masturbation or the sexual encounter with the maid. The psychiatrist's response to the latter is simply: 'That's all right'. Third, while we have a rather superficial account here – although a lot of dialogue is reproduced, presumably from the psychiatrist's notes – this was not a superficial process. Dick was seen over a long period in what appears to have been numerous sessions. Fourth, the psychiatrist's approach prefigures that which becomes much more common in post-war child guidance, namely leading the patient to an understanding of his purported illness rather than prescriptively telling him, or his parents, what to do. Of course we have a partial account here focused on the role of the psychiatrist and it may well be that the PSW was attempting simultaneously to alter parental attitudes. But, if so, she did not appear to succeed. And, in any event, it is the mother in particular who is seen as the author of her child's misfortune. Fifth, the mother's shortcomings as a parent are partly because of her own emotional difficulties although it is accepted that she did not act through ill-will or malice. The issue of parent blaming, and more particularly mother blaming, is returned to below but a comment by Jones on contemporary American child guidance is especially pertinent here as it fits one aspect of Dick's case almost exactly. Mothers perceived as domineering wives, Jones writes, allegedly 'created spineless husbands who stayed away from their children to avoid confrontations and thus deprived their children of necessary guidance'.[44]

Our second case comes from London and the case notes of the PSW Robina Addis.[45] This particular young girl, age unspecified but pubescent (and probably close to school-leaving age), was referred for stealing and truancy. She had been seen the previous year by Burt whose report indicated that her emotional instability could be attributed to 'heredity, lack of home control and puberty' and that her appearance was 'unattractive and dirty'. Among the potential solutions was removal from the home but the family would not countenance this. Between seeing Burt and the girl's present referral the LCC Care Committee worker had given up her home visits as 'useless'.

At the initial case conference it was noted that the patient was one of three surviving children of seven and presently lived with her father, her 21-year-old sister and a niece aged two-and-a-half years. Her mother had died two years previously and was reported to have been 'unstable and of violent temper' and the household, located in slum property but 'kept spick and span', was run by the elder sister. The family dynamics were that the elder sister resented the patient's failure to help with household maintenance. There was little domestic control, with the father, an unemployed dock worker, being 'easy going, affectionate and kindly'. The infant was spoiled. The father was not especially concerned about the patient's stealing and supported her ambition to leave school and get a job.

The girl had scored well on her IQ test, 116. The psychiatrist suggested that her exaggerated nonchalance was an attempt to cover 'adolescent emotionality'. At present she was not 'readily amenable to psycho-therapy' but that with suitable employment she would be likely to adjust well. This case conference concluded that it was best for now that the girl stayed at home but that she should leave home at 14 and get a job and that 'attempts should be made to get some older person from a club or girl guides really interested in her'.

It was against this background that Addis made her home visit some six weeks later. By this time it had been noted that the patient had 'taken up with a wild lot of girls' at her new school and that she 'goes with the school boys too' although her sister thought this was not anything to worry about. Addis observed that the patient was 'extremely wayward and irresponsible', that she was unwashed and that she showed physical signs of having been out late the previous evening. As to the father, he seemed 'vaguely distressed' about his younger daughter, threatened to 'thrash' her if she carried on as at present and even suggested that she might go to a foster home. Addis concluded that he had no control over the girl and that it was 'unlikely that repeated interviews could change his attitude' – he could be helped 'only in practical ways'. This took an immediate form in that the girl had the opportunity to participate in a charitably supported country holiday but was refusing to go unless she got more dresses. A further complication arose with the arrival of a neighbour who told Addis that the patient had one breast more developed than the other. The neighbour had offered to take the girl to the hospital and on her refusal 'warned her that it might have to be cut off'. Faced with this somewhat challenging situation the PSW suggested that the girl have a physical examination and, rather vaguely, that individual attention might be helpful (the patient would have nothing to do with clubs). Addis also noted the possibility of the home breaking up and that the charity organizing the country holiday might be approached for assistance with clothing. Finally, she recommended that, if at all possible, the eldest daughter should see a psychiatrist, presumably on the basis that it was she who was doing everything in the household and consequently showing signs of strain.

What immediate comments can we make about this case? First, we have a child who at least in terms of intellectual endowment is normal. Second, although socio-economic circumstances are alluded to they are not given any weight in assessing the origins of the girl's problems. Third, we have a mother who is absent through death but who had, purportedly, her own mental health problems. The father, meanwhile, is unable to control the girl and despite his initial characterization as affectionate and indifferent to her misdemeanours, by the time of Addis's visit is displaying a changed attitude towards his daughter. Revealingly, the PSW places no faith in any attempt to alter him suggesting instead that his eldest daughter receive psychiatric counselling. Addis thus effectively concedes the household to the latter's control. Fourth, the implied sexual misbehaviour is not addressed. Finally, Addis resorts to a very 'traditional' social work approach by appealing to a charity for support to enable the patient to go on her country holiday.

Another of Addis's cases threw up a different series of problems. This concerned a schoolboy – exact age not specified – who was proving slow to learn, had poor coordination, did not get on with other children and was restless and lacking in concentration. In large part this was explained by the child's low IQ. He was almost, in the language of the time, mentally deficient. But his problems also had a temperamental dimension and 'the irritability, tempers and ready tears show emotional strain'. A 'glance at the home situation', Addis continued, 'gives an impression of tension'. The mother was 'dreamy, unsociable' and more irritated than the father by their son. The PSW inferred that the mother's falls during pregnancy suggested attempts to induce a miscarriage and the boy's preschool problems – slow development and not being toilet trained until five – too would have done little to engender a sense in him of being wanted. The father was a 'sociable person' who, since the mother would not accompany him in his frequent outings to British Legion clubs, 'takes out her vivacious friend'. He was more tolerant of the boy although he admitted to losing his temper with him. The parents, Addis suggested, were dissatisfied with each other which perhaps led them to having little 'capacity for giving affection to a child'.[46]

Treatment would therefore have to be based on 'relieving tension in the home' and to encouraging the child to adapt to school life and to 'stand up for himself'. The father was 'certainly the most important person to re-educate' but also probably the most difficult as he was happy with his present lifestyle. The mother would best be dealt with by the father paying her more attention since '[n]othing is so becoming as admiration'. This in turn would encourage her to take 'a pride in her appearance' which would be 'more durable than if merely stimulated by the social worker' and thereby 'subject to collapse if snubbed by the Father for whom the attraction was intended'.

Here we have a rather different case in that the patient is of low IQ and this is viewed as contributing to his troubles. Nonetheless, the child's problems are also seen as having a psychological and emotional basis deriving from familial dynamics and in particular the lack of parental affection for the patient, especially on the mother's part. So while the child is to be, essentially, told to pull his socks up, it is the parents who are to be the prime focus of attention. This was to involve, it is assumed, the PSW encouraging the father to pay more attention to his wife and her appearance, perhaps at the expense of her 'vivacious friend'. Again we find the emotional dysfunctionality of at least one of the parents, and certainly of the relationship between them, crucially shaping the child's own mental well-being. What we also find, though, is a normative assessment of how the malfunctioning spousal relationship should be addressed.

Our next case comes from a famous article by Bowlby relatively early in his career and based on 150 case studies from the London Clinic. This relates to Sheila C., a four-and-a-half-year-old referred for 'screaming fits and destructiveness'. Sheila, an only child, had a mental age of 6 – she was an intelligent girl – but was highly resistant to going to school. For Bowlby it was clear from the first interview that this patient was neurotic. He attributed her screaming fits at school to her having been told off and concluded there was, overall, much evidence to show a 'strong sense of guilt which she was trying to evade and to get reassurance against'. Sheila's hostility and guilt in turn derived from her mother's attitude and treatment of her. Mrs C. – a woman of 'obviously irritable temperament' in contrast to her more easy-going husband – had given birth shortly after marriage and the pregnancy had not been planned. The mother looked after Sheila during the day and was jealous of her husband's use of his leisure time away from the home. An intelligent woman, she acknowledged that her daughter's problems might be due to her not wanting the baby in the first place although this self-knowledge did not stop her slapping the child when irritated by her. But there was more to it. Mrs C. herself had felt rejected when a child and resentful of her stepsister. After a 'considerable number of interviews' Bowlby succeeded in making the mother understand the source of her problem and 'her attitude to Sheila improved very considerably, with the result that Sheila's symptoms almost disappeared'. But the girl remained a 'neurotic child', having 'introjected her mother's condemning attitude very fully' although it was possible that the changed maternal attitude would, 'over a period of years', help Sheila 'back to normality'. At the very least things would not get any worse.[47]

As in a number of our case studies we have here, first, a situation where maternal affection is purportedly withheld at a crucial stage in the child's development and the consequent addressing of the child's problem through the emotional education of the mother. Again, this is a labour-intensive process. We also have another instance of problems in the childhood of one generation leading to problems in the next, an issue with which Bowlby was much concerned. And although in this case Bowlby does not appear to make much of it, the fact that Sheila is an only child is worth commenting on as this too was thought by many child guidance practitioners to be especially problematic. Indeed any parent whose child was shy, highly intelligent and had no siblings was deemed to have serious concerns. Finally, there is the rather gloomy prognosis that the patient will take a long time to recover, if she ever does. However much Mrs C. has changed, this is not of itself enough.

If withholding affection could lead to maladjustment so too could its opposite – over-affection or spoiling. In *Mother and Child*, Dr Levinson of the East

London clinic described Leonard's case. This 6-year-old boy had been referred for night terrors, enuresis, fear of dark places and 'generally difficult behaviour'. He had an average IQ and the family circumstances were comfortable. His mother told the psychiatrist that Leonard had been a 'model child' until the birth of his sister three years earlier. On the mother's own admission she had spoiled Leonard prior to this, but had not forewarned him of his sister's arrival. He subsequently became extremely jealous and clung to his mother. The boy also became physically ill as a consequence of his continual crying, developing a hernia which necessitated a stay in hospital. During this period his mother did 'everything possible to give in to the child in an attempt to pacify him', but after the operation bed-wetting and screaming attacks started. Investigation had shown, then, that the 'first step to his neurosis was the over-affection displayed by the mother, which prepared the way for future mischief'. There was a further problem in the shape of the father. The latter, while affectionate towards other members of the family was markedly not so with Leonard. Levinson, perhaps having studied Freud, concluded that the two were in rivalry for the mother's affection and that the child undoubtedly 'harboured a death wish of the father'. It also became apparent that the father was of 'the infantile, emotional type' and that it was he who was 'in urgent need of child guidance'. However the mother, once she understood the situation, proved to be a 'good ally' in terms of treatment and consequently 'great improvement was effected in the child's condition in a very short time'.[48]

Leonard thus appears to have been the victim of a three-pronged emotional attack despite his otherwise normal circumstances. Spoiled by his mother – she sees him initially as a 'model' child by which is presumably meant compliant – and jealous of the birth of his sister, he is also deprived of affection from his father. Other profound psychological forces are also at work, notably the boy's rivalry with his father for the mother's affection and his death wish towards the former. The trenchant critique of the father is rather unusual in this period – fathers are generally absent physically, emotionally or both – but it is also revealing that once more the means of resolving the situation is through the mother, suitably counselled as to how to restore domestic emotional equilibrium.

Again from the East London Clinic, but this time from the PSW's perspective, we have the case of a 5-year-old boy. Once more we encounter a highly intelligent child, IQ 135. He and his mother had been deserted by the father and, having been comfortably off, were now 'reduced to living in one room'. The mother, a fairly well-educated woman, was in a 'tense emotional state' and this was having an obvious impact on the boy, who was developing 'peculiar mannerisms'. The PSW's solution was, first, to arrange the child's removal to a boarding school 'for the children of working people'. This appeared to work, with the boy performing well and visiting his mother in the school holidays. The mother herself proved more intractable. She had sold up what remained of her home and obtained a post in domestic service. In her emotionally overwrought state, however, she was unable to adjust to her new environment and gave up her job 'at the first trifling difficulty'. Another social work intervention ensued. A place at a convalescent home was arranged with the help of a charity, after two months of which 'she appeared to be much restored in mind and body'. Another domestic service post was obtained and she now seemed to be 'a happier and more stabilised individual'.[49]

Three points stand out here. First, we see the removal of the child from the home. This was something which was generally, and increasingly as time went on, avoided in child guidance practice. However, in this particular case such was mother's condition that modifying her behaviour was out of the question, at least in the short term. Second, we once more observe a focus on the mother as the object of attention. Although it is acknowledged that her socio-economic circumstances have been drastically reduced, and while the social work interventions can be seen as partially addressing this issue, nonetheless it is the mother's 'tense emotional state' which is doing the damage. Finally, we again see more 'traditional' social work practices coming into play – a respectable woman is found a respectable job and charitable aid is called upon.

Our last case comes from the Edinburgh Catholic Clinic and concerns a teenage girl, exact age unspecified.[50] The psychiatrist's report started with an interview with the child's stepmother, a 'bright intelligent woman' genuinely anxious to do her best by the patient. In this vein the stepmother did find some positive things to say about the girl – for instance she did not steal from the home and was good at housework. The patient's early history included her mother's death and a consequent shifting between various relatives, none of whom, by the stepmother's account, gave her any training. Consequently, when the stepmother arrived on the scene the child had 'no proper underclothing, her head and body were verminous and she used to wet the bed at nights'. The patient was also suspected of masturbation and the stepmother described a series of meetings, some three years previously, between the child and an unidentified man. Again on the issue of sexual misbehaviour the patient had been among a group of girls caught at school with notes 'containing disgusting and filthy language and referring to things of a sexual nature'. The child was also lazy, quick tempered, never spoke to either the stepmother or the father and was 'very stupid'. The interview with the father was hardly more upbeat. Although cooperative, he gave 'the impression of having little real affection' for his daughter and 'seemed rather anxious to be rid of her'. He too referred to the child's 'filthy habits' and found her 'so stupid she could not understand anything'.

There are, in addition to those with the stepmother and the father, two recorded interviews with the child herself. At the first of these the patient – 'a thin, dark-haired child, manner quiet but not shy' – gave an account of her life, initially answering questions freely and openly. When it came to sexual matters she acknowledged discussions with other girls from an early age. But, the psychiatrist noted, she 'would not tell me what other girls had told her and at one point she became rather emotional and began to weep'. The psychiatrist sought to reassure her, explaining that 'I would help her to understand anything she wanted to know and that she could ask me any questions she liked'. This appeared to work in that at least from the psychiatrist's perspective they parted on friendly terms.

At the second meeting the patient confessed to disliking her parents but would not say why. She admitted to masturbation, that she had done it for a long time, that she had learned to do it by herself and that she 'could not help doing it'. Again in the psychiatrist's words the child seemed 'to be frightened and inclined to be tearful when we discussed this and I think it probable that she has been scolded and threatened at home for this habit'. Summing up, the child's low IQ – borderline deficiency – was recorded as well as the fact that this might 'be accompanied by an innate weakness in ability to inhibit her instincts and to develop aesthetic and moral sentiments'. Her early training had been 'deplorable'. She had probably gained a considerable amount of sexual knowledge and 'possibly sexual experience' at a young age and this had 'stimulated an inordinate curiosity in the subject'. Finally, the girl appeared to have a 'deep-rooted feeling of resentment against her parents'. This might be justified in that she may have heard herself described as 'dirty, useless, stupid etc' or might be based on persecution fantasy 'of the sort that mental defectives were inclined to indulge in'. Indeed some of her habits may have been 'an attempt to revenge herself on her parents', something which needed further investigation.

What immediate points can we make about this unfortunate child? First, like the first of Addis's cases the mother has died, the ultimate form of maternal absence. In this case, though, there is not even a suggestion that the father shows any affection for his daughter – on the contrary. Her experience of lack of affection from early childhood is thus clearly seen as formative. Second, the issue of sexual knowledge and practice again arises. More than this, there is a strong sense in this case of sexual abuse. Third, we again see a psychiatrist acting in a way which encouraged the child and which thus at least allowed for some move, on the latter's part, towards self-knowledge. But unlike Dick this is a patient with a low IQ, which not only complicates the emotional chaos she finds herself in, but also leads the psychiatrist to see it as possibly resulting in fantasy formation and the use of particular behaviours to – albeit possibly with justification – revenge herself on her father and mother substitute. In short, her low intelligence combined with affectionless parenting has led to the patient's present predicament.

Before moving to more general observations it is worth stressing that, as individuals and professionals, there can be little doubt that psychiatrists, psychologists and PSWs saw themselves as operating in the child's interests. Similarly, it seems probable that some children benefitted from child guidance interventions, if not necessarily thanks to child guidance's underpinning assumptions. Whether this was true of parents, and particularly mothers, is another matter. So what occurred in and around child guidance clinics deserves historically critical attention and this is returned to in the concluding chapter. But what broad issues arise from our case studies?

First, while reference was made in some instances to socio-economic circumstances, these were not seen as determining factors in the child's problems. The existence of comfortably off or middle-class patients simply seemed to reinforce this claim. Second, it is clear that their professional training notwithstanding, PSWs would on occasion resort to more 'traditional' social work methods, often in this pre-welfare state era involving appeals to charities. Third, there is the question of child sexuality. On the issue of masturbation child guidance professionals took a relatively relaxed attitude, only seeing it as a problem or worthy of prolonged comment if deemed excessive (as in the last case). This was commendable since, as Hera Cook points out, even more 'progressive' parents in this era remained deeply upset by this sexual practice. Such a professional attitude was almost certainly shaped by Freud's view that masturbation was something engaged in by most children and adolescents.[51] On sexual abuse it is revealing that Bowlby, in his 1987 recollections of the early days of child guidance, lamented 'our complete ignorance of either the occurrence or the ill-effects of physical and sexual abuse.'[52] The evasion of this issue may have been due to the arguments of psychiatrists such as Freud, initially at least, that children's reports of sexual encounters with adults were fantasy rather than fact.

Fourth, it is notable that for all its scientific aspirations child guidance practitioners were not immune from making normative judgements. It is, of course, easy to understand that Dick's father might be 'slightly sentimental' or his mother 'somewhat hard, undemonstrative' but these are hardly precise clinical assessments. Similarly, Burt's description of the girl subsequently seen by Addis as 'unattractive and dirty' does not really move the diagnosis along. And the notion that the problems encountered in Addis's second case could be resolved by the mother making herself more attractive might be seen as all too typical of the time, but also as precisely illuminating the point that attitudes to behaviour are socially and historically constructed.

Finally, there is the issue of where responsibility for the child's maladjustment lay. Unsurprisingly, given the underlying premise that difficulties arose primarily from problematic familial relationships, it was deemed to be with the parents. This could take the form of tensions between one or both parents and the child, deriving from emotional or psychological parental malfunction or between the parents, with their unhappiness transmitting itself to the child. Either way, there was in addition the possibility of a generational effect, unhappiness in the parents leading to unhappiness in the child and so on. We discuss the issue of tensions between parents further below.

But it is also important to identify another dimension of attributing responsibility to the parent. For in most cases dealt with by child guidance clinics it was the mother or the mother substitute who was seen as the pivotal figure. Even in the second case cited above, where the mother was dead and no stepmother present, it was the elder sister who ran the home and who was recommended for psychiatric help. Mothers might be over-affectionate, under-affectionate or have withdrawn affection and any of these would result in child maladjustment. Of course on one level this focus on the mother simply reflected the contemporary gender division of labour. Many men worked long hours while for mothers, at least of younger children, their place remained very much as homemakers. Nonetheless while the language of 'blame' was often, although far from always, eschewed, there is a strong case that what social interventions such as child guidance did was, in effect, to blame the mother while seeing her simultaneously as the means whereby her child's problems might be resolved. The mother, to put it another way, was subjected to treatment as much as the child and this is one clear message of our case studies. Discussing American child guidance, Jones remarks that motherhood developed a particular status both as a cause of juvenile misbehavior and as itself the subject of medical scrutiny. British practice mirrors this trend and almost certainly drew upon it. Jones attributes maternal status in part to the exertion of professional authority over mothers, not only by male psychiatrists but also by female PSWs.[53] Plant, meanwhile and again discussing the US, notes that from the 1920s 'new and more psychologically oriented critiques of motherhood emerged, and mother-blaming expanded to encompass middle-class as well as poor mothers.'[54] Once more, this throws light on the similar British experience.

Problem Parents and Clinic Outcomes

What more, then, can we say about the problems of problem parents? In the introductory chapter we noted MacCalman's 1937 plea for his 'visionary dream' that a 'vast system of parent education' be realized. The clear implication here was that parents were presently uneducated and hence that older ideas about, in particular, maternal instinct as an adequate guide to childrearing were no longer acceptable. Other child guidance psychiatrists similarly looked to parents as, if not the whole problem, then at least as having a significant part to play in their child's mental distress. Moodie commented that parents 'often feel that they are the cause of their children's difficulties, and in so far as they are responsible for their training and upbringing, this is true'. He sought, though, to distinguish between responsibility and blame and it was not his clinic's 'practice to ascribe guilt to parents'. 'The average parent', Moodie continued, 'especially if his child presents problems of behaviour, is ready to help in treatment if the principles to be followed are presented clearly and rationally to him. This is where the methods of Child Guidance surpass other methods'.[55] The purported distinction between responsibility and guilt echoes that between factual and moral blame encountered above in the case of Dick's parents.

Burns remarked that it was certainly an exaggeration to say that there were no problem children, only problem parents. Many other factors were involved in the creation of maladjustment. Nonetheless there were certain circumstances in which parental neuroses had to be addressed and the two volunteer psychiatrists which his clinic had by this time acquired had enabled the 'treatment of parents at the Clinic'. This had a number of advantages, foremost amongst which was the 'unification and coordination in the treatment of the family situation'.[56] Around the same time Burns asked to be relieved of some of his official activities outside of child guidance as he was 'increasingly anxious to have time for the psycho-therapy of adults as well as children'. After consultation with the Board of Education this was agreed to.[57]

This was acknowledgement of the increasing focus on the parent and the Board later clarified the issue. It was, its officials suggested, in agreement with Birmingham Corporation that a 'certain amount of psychological investigation of parents is an essential feature of Child Guidance work, and forms part of the treatment of the child'. It was therefore permissible for LEAs to carry out such work. What was outwith their remit was the treatment of parents separately from their children although it was suggested that were volunteers to carry this out there would be no opposition from the Board – the issue was therefore one of finance and the legal position of Education Authorities. Birmingham thus took the view that psychological investigation of parents could take place 'provided this is done concurrently with the treatment of the children and does not involve special sessions or appointments for parents as distinct from children'.[58] This was a bureaucratic endorsement of something that was, in fact, fundamental to child guidance – that a child's maladjustment was generated in the context of the family and that the problem thus lay in the final resort with one or both parents.

But of course parents, most parents, were misguided or wrongheaded rather than in need of any serious psychiatric intervention. As we shall see in chapter 6, MacCalman was in a post-war speech even to suggest that a bad parent was better than no parent at all. What parents therefore required, as Moodie's comments suggest, was guidance and we have noted the role of non-specialist outlets such as *Mother and Child* in spreading and popularizing the child guidance message. One area where this was particularly pertinent was discipline. As again we shall see in chapter 6, the place of the child in post-war society led to child guidance commentary on the degree of 'freedom' which it should be accorded. But this had been a concern from the outset albeit not articulated in the language of social reconstruction which prevailed in the 1940s. So what were the concerns around freedom and discipline in the interwar period, given the strains of modernity and broader socio-economic and political instability?

Moodie in particular devoted much attention to this issue. He told the Liverpool Child Guidance Council in 1933 that society was 'suffering from a lack of control and guidance in the bringing up of children – an epidemic of what people call freedom, but which is not freedom, but licence'.[59] Readers of *Mother and Child* were advised that they would 'get the best out of their children and make them happy' – happiness again – if they were 'sensible and restrained in the exercise both of authority and kindness'. Under certain circumstances this would require punishment, the need for which Moodie had no doubt. 'All social life', he suggested, 'depends on discipline', although it had to be appropriate to the misdemeanour and should not be administered as it so often was 'as a relief for the feelings of the adult'.[60] What we once more see, as with the approach to masturbation and in the more general view that emotions should be expressed but not overexpressed, was a sort of 'middle way' between overindulgence and excessive strictness. Moderation in both childhood behaviour and in parenting was thus the key to individual, familial and ultimately social integration and stability.

What were the outcomes of these clinical approaches? Revealingly, this was something about which child guidance practitioners were rather defensive. Burns not only noted the difficulty of translating 'facts and estimates' into hard data due to the lack of 'fixed standards' but also that, 'for what they are worth', results from his own clinic showed 'approximately the same kind of results as reported from other clinics'.[61] This was hardly a ringing claim for clinical success. A few years later he commented that it was 'often said that Child Guidance is still in its experimental stage, and that only time will tell whether it has any real value'. In response, he suggested that 'any art or science which deals with human beings – whether it be politics, education, or medicine – will always be in an experimental stage, with constant new theories and developments, often re-discovering ancient truths under new forms'.[62] Moodie made the similarly downbeat remark that, with respect to the London Clinic, its results 'compare favourably with those obtained in other branches of medicine'.[63]

As with definition and aetiological classification, though, clinics tried to give some sense of outcomes. That attached to Guy's Hospital reported that for 1930, 40 per cent of its patients were 'much improved', with 17 per cent 'improved' and 27 per cent 'unchanged'. Allocated to the same categories in 1933 were, respectively, 16, 48 and 15 per cent of patients with a further 6 per cent 'worse'.[64] These differences might be explained by different types of patient – which is unlikely – or a refinement of classificatory techniques. Either way, such categories can be seen as less than clinically exact. At Birmingham in the late 1930s some 75 per cent of patients were discharged as 'sufficiently adjusted or improved', In a typical

Burns qualification the report continued that the 'test however is one of quality than of quantity'. It was

> more important to be able to point to a small number of cases, showing very serious symptoms of maladjustment, who have become well adjusted in themselves and to their surrounding, and have remained so for a number of months or years after treatment, than to be able to claim a percentage of total results.[65]

Nonetheless, lack of clarity and precision in terms of definition, classification and outcomes was to leave child guidance open to criticism by those sceptical of its methods and claims.

Contemporary Critiques

So here we might note contemporary criticism from individuals and bodies not directly involved in child guidance provision. The Birmingham educationalist C.W. Valentine agreed that clinics had done some good. But he also counselled against making 'fallacious inferences' from such success, not least that the 'peculiar methods of a particular Clinic' must necessarily be the main cause of any 'cure'. Valentine correctly pointed out that different clinics used different techniques with similar results and even, citing evidence from the child guidance movement itself, that the 'recovery rates' of 'treated and untreated' groups were 'regrettably similar'.[66] On the question of whether children might recover with or without the help of child guidance, an LCC committee made a similar point. It had been claimed that of the cases referred to the London Clinic some 45 per cent had been successfully dealt with. It was, though, 'undoubtedly' the case that in certain instances 'the root of the trouble and a recommendation for treatment could have been reached without the elaborate technique of child guidance'.[67] And the Feversham Committee, while broadly supportive and acknowledging that the majority of its patients had been 'cured' or 'relieved or improved', nonetheless added the serious qualification that little could be said of the 'success or otherwise of the efforts made by the child guidance clinics ... to treat individual children, for no scientific method has been devised for measuring the results of treatment'.[68]

From a very different perspective there were those who agreed that children might need psychiatric treatment while rejecting the child guidance approach. The psychiatrist John Rickman, a follower of Melanie Klein, contributed a preface to a volume significantly entitled *On the Bringing up of Children*. Here Rickman noted that Freud had created a new scientific 'instrument of research' in the form of analysis and this had given 'greater definition and exactness' to the insights of child welfare and education. Analysis had shown too that the growth of the child's mind was a 'far more complicated process than was once supposed'. Hence 'much harm may be done' if a 'method of upbringing is adopted which

underestimates the complexities'. In a key passage Rickman argued that one conclusion drawn 'by those who have not grasped the real implications of the "new
psychology"' was that 'if a child were properly brought up he would have no
serious difficulties, and that the prevalence of nervous troubles is proof that parents are always doing the wrong thing to their offspring'. This was both untrue
and a disservice to children and parents alike. It obscured the 'importance of the
child's own intricate mental activities', thus viewing him as 'a piece of inactive
plastic material'.[69] It is difficult not to see this as an attack on the child guidance
approach and not least in the latter's propensity to look to parents for both cause
of and solution to their child's problems. Rickman's critique is also worth seeing
in the context of a number of the issues raised previously: child guidance's desire
to see itself as 'scientific'; by contrast its advocacy of the 'commonsense conversation' between psychiatrist and child patient; and its belief in the plasticity and
relative shallowness of the child's mind.

Conclusion

This chapter has engaged with child guidance issues concerning measurement,
diagnosis and treatment. These have included how to determine the crucial
concept of 'normalcy' and how to assess the efficacy of clinical engagements.
It has been suggested that problems in such areas, often acknowledged at the
time, nonetheless cast doubt on child guidance's claims to scientific precision
and laid it open to attack by those with varying degrees of lack of sympathy for
child guidance and its methods. These were issues which were not to go away.
We have also examined even less easily defined emotional states such as shyness
and happiness. The former, it has been argued, was a further example of how
a behavioural characteristic could be placed under the child guidance gaze for
no reason other than that it was thought to be in some way socially unsatisfactory. And we have gained some sense of what actually went on in child guidance
practice. Crucially, this tended to shift the focus of engagement away from the
child and to the parents and in particular the mother. Mothers came to be seen
as one of the key contributory factors in child maladjustment and, while under
the direction of child guidance professionals, the means of returning the child
patient to normalcy. Again, such issues were to continue to resonate and to have
longer-term implications. Our next step is to analyse child guidance in wartime.

5 CHILD GUIDANCE IN WARTIME

Introduction

British child guidance had, by 1939, grown in terms of the number of clinics and the number of patients referred. Although the spread was uneven, recognition by the Board of Education and the Commonwealth Fund's continuing support had resulted in the establishment of clinics both in London and in other parts of the country. In financial terms these were maintained by voluntary donations, local authority support, indirect CGC subsidies or a mixture of all three. The child guidance message was also being spread by way of popular journals and by the educational activities of practitioners and supporters. The experience of clinic patients too has been examined as have concepts such as normalcy and happiness.

In this chapter we examine child guidance in wartime. We focus first on the significance of evacuation for child guidance's development. The former derived not only from the experience of evacuation but also by way of, for example, surveys undertaken to assess its impact. Such surveys, although differing in terms of methodology, nonetheless reinforced the idea that the child's home environment was crucial to its mental well-being and that most maladjustment found among evacuees in fact pre-dated removal from the family home. By and large, then, evacuation highlighted existing problems rather than actually creating them. We examine too the continuing growth of child guidance provision, the organizational and economic constraints of wartime notwithstanding, and the actual practice of child guidance under such challenging conditions. Finally, we look at how child guidance advocates saw its further development once the war was over.

The Evacuation Process

By the late 1930s the authorities had prepared for evacuation from urban areas deemed to be at risk from enemy bombing.[1] The country was divided into three zones: the Sending Areas, the parts of the country thought to be threatened by aerial attack; Reception Areas, areas considered unlikely to be bombed and which were often predominantly rural; and Neutral Areas. The official schemes were to be voluntary and primarily involved children. Underpinning these preparations were the widespread beliefs that war was inevitable and that large-scale aerial bombing would immediately ensue, that such bombing would have a profound impact on the civilian population both physically and psychologically and that evacuees might be absent from home for a prolonged period. Ultimately, there were to be three waves of evacuation, the first and most significant in terms of its wider social impact taking place immediately at the onset of war.

Prior to the conflict two developments of particular relevance to child guidance took place. First, it was agreed that PSWs would be included among the Reserved Occupations.[2] This was later to be further reinforced, as evacuation was under way, by a Ministry of Health Circular which stressed the 'desirability of using staff experienced in child guidance' with difficult children in the Reception Areas, of itself an acknowledgement of the potential contribution of child guidance to children's mental well-being.[3] Second, the Mental Health Emergency Committee was formed in 1938 in the wake of the Feversham Report and in response to the mental health issues which it was thought would arise during the impending conflict. The Committee merged the CGC, the Central Association for Mental Welfare and the National Council for Mental Hygiene.[4] In May 1939 the Emergency Committee wrote to the Board of Education arguing that any emotional disturbances arising from war would impact especially hard on children. In addition, it was likely that many child guidance clinics, such as those in London, would be closed. This would present a particularly difficult problem for those in the Reception Areas since they would be faced with 'so mixed a group, containing, as it will, defective, dull, and problem children, as well as those maladjusted in their new environment'. It was thus a matter of urgency that 'skilled and experienced workers whose Child Guidance Clinics may be closed should not be scattered, but should be available as far as possible as corporate units for this important and difficult work'.[5]

When war came, 1.4 million children were evacuated, with children under school age accompanied by their mothers. This was a huge movement of people and, in particular, children. So, for instance, some 400,000 unaccompanied school children left London.[6] Evacuees came overwhelmingly from inner-city, working-class neighbourhoods. Although the evacuation which took place in 1939 for the most part lasted only a very short time, its impact was huge. This was in part because of the condition and behaviour of the evacuated children. Even a relatively sympathetic report recorded that from the host communities' standpoint problems such as bed-wetting were widely resented, with other behavioural issues including wilful vandalism. As noted in the introductory chapter, this particular report then went on to suggest that the evacuation experience demonstrated the need for greater child guidance provision in Scotland, deemed at present to be only 'in its infancy'.[7] Such a conclusion was commonplace in accounts of evacuation as well as being part of a wider call for enhanced child guidance services.

Evacuation and Child Guidance

How, then, did child guidance supporters respond to evacuation and what conclusions did they draw? In the late 1940s, by which point child guidance was part of the welfare state, Moodie published a revised edition of his book on child psychiatry aimed primarily at GPs. The war had, he observed, certainly created problems for children. These were due to, inter alia, the absence of fathers and a decline in moral standards. But in general his book would make no detailed reference to the war since 'it produced no particular or unusual differences' as far as British children were concerned. Of those who had directly experienced bombing few 'suffered any ill effects'. With respect to evacuation for some it 'was a terrible experience, but these were the over-protected, the insecure, and the unstable'.[8]

In his retrospective survey of schoolchildren's health during the war the Ministry of Education's CMO noted that evacuation in 1939 had 'brought forcibly to light the presence and the problems of children who were psychologically maladjusted'. Some of these had already been identified and special provision made for them. However the great majority of children found to be troublesome had given no sign of this, at least publicly, prior to evacuation. 'This was not surprising', he continued, 'for most of their maladjustment had not been exhibited or seen during school hours. Evacuation merely brought to public notice troubles previously only known in their own homes'.[9] None of this was to play down evacuation's significance for child guidance – the CMO's comments came from a chapter in his report entitled 'Child Guidance', clearly implying a relationship between the evacuation experience and enhanced child guidance services. The impact of evacuation lay not in creating maladjustment but in shining light on a pre-existing problem. An especially gloomy picture, though, had been painted as evacuation began to take place in autumn 1939.

In September 1939 Miller and Bowlby attended a meeting at the Board of Education. Bowlby was to further participate in debates about evacuation and its lessons for child mental health services and, in an almost uncanny piece of timing, 1939 had seen the publication of his co-authored book, *Personal Aggressiveness and War*. This paid considerable attention to aggression in children and drew upon Bowlby's experience at the London Clinic as well as on the work of Susan Isaacs, whom he knew from his time as a doctoral student under Burt.[10] Underpinning this work, Ben Mayhew argues, was that psychological intervention by the state was necessary 'for the maintenance of the peace and the active cooperation with others that would make possible the division of labour and the creation of an affluent society'.[11] The wider implications of psychological health once more come to the fore here. The more immediate context of Bowlby and Miller's visit was the widespread belief in pre-war psychiatric circles that the impending conflict would bring a greater number of psychiatric than physical casualties and proposals for mobile teams of psychiatrists and mobile child guidance clinics.[12]

At the Board of Education meeting, Miller and Bowlby claimed that problems would arise as a result of evacuation. More than this, there was the issue of evacuated children who were already maladjusted and who had possibly even already attended child guidance clinics. This latter group posed particular difficulties and special provision might be necessary. Bowlby, it was recorded, had raised such matters with Evelyn Fox who in turn had arranged for a group of volunteers, including some twenty to thirty PSWs, to investigate conditions where London evacuees were billeted. Looking to the future, Bowlby argued that the service he envisaged for evacuated children 'was not designed solely to meet the present difficulties but would be largely preventive, and the expenditure on it would be a wise precaution'. While older children might be the cause of immediate problems 'there were very serious psychological dangers attendant on the removal of young children from their mothers, and these would not begin to manifest for some time'. Bowlby's interest in infants and in the long-term implications of separation is clearly evident here. His own experience – he was here clearly alluding to his research into the psychological origins of delinquency – suggested that such children might become delinquents and that separation could lead to 'large scale social maladaptation'. He would thus prefer to 'see young children whose mothers were not evacuated remain with them in the danger zones rather than face the unknown problems of a parting for as long as three years'.[13] Bowlby had already publicly made similar points to fellow child guidance clinic practitioners in 1939.[14]

Bowlby was clearly articulating the then-prevalent belief that evacuees would be away from home for a long period. More remarkable is his assertion that it was better for at least younger children to face the physical dangers attendant upon staying in threatened urban areas rather than face the psychological dangers of separation. This was an argument made on more than one occasion. In a book aimed at an American audience Anne St Loe Strachey cited an anonymous psychiatrist to this effect.[15] In a slightly less dramatic way Anna Freud and Dorothy Burlingham, child psychologists who ran the famous Hampstead nurseries, noted in 1942 that 'evacuation under the present conditions is as upsetting as bombing itself'.[16]

Whatever Bowlby and Miller's aspirations, central government faced problems. The Board of Education, in correspondence shortly after the meeting with the two psychiatrists, noted that ideally Reception Areas should have a child psychiatrist's services to identify 'the real problem child (as apart from the merely naughty or homesick child in an unsuitable billet)'. However only in a few did there exist 'any arrangements for child guidance or similar work', a situation compounded by the current lack of suitably trained psychiatrists. In addition other aspects of evacuation had been preoccupying those in the Reception Areas. Nonetheless it was now time, the official concluded, to talk again to Fox and other interested parties 'with a view to ascertaining the number of qualified workers who are likely to be available, the terms on which their services could be obtained, and the best way of distributing them among the reception areas'.[17] Such comments illustrate both the limitations of existing child guidance provision and the perceived relationship between evacuation and the need for such services. It was also noted that despite earlier concerns in late October 1939 more than half of the recognized child guidance clinics in England and Wales remained open – essentially all of those outside London and Southampton.[18] The flagship London Clinic was to remain closed for the rest of the war although its training and clinical functions were returned in 1943 to, respectively, the Woodside Hospital and the Middlesex Hospital.[19] The CGC evacuated to Cambridge and opened a small clinical unit there.[20] It was here that Bowlby met the social reformer Margery Fry a decade later, who was instrumental in the publishing of *Child Care and the Growth of Love*.[21]

Analysis of evacuation's impact and its implications for child guidance also came from those directly involved at or near its front line. Liverpool's evacuees featured strongly in the backlash against the process. Reflecting on the city's experience, the child guidance clinic's Director observed that removal from home might psychologically 'have a disastrous effect, especially where a child already has an emotional insecurity, arising from some unsatisfactory factor in the parent–child relationship'. Even those whose 'security is fundamentally firm' might experience 'great shock' and all this suggested a probable need for child guidance greater than under 'normal conditions'. There were 'several aspects of present-day conditions which foreshadow an increase in the nervous and behaviour disorders of children'. These included evacuation and disruption to education. More generally, and echoing Moodie's comments about the absence of fathers and the slackening of discipline, the report argued that

> war conditions must bring an increasing disturbance in the family constitution, the absence in many instances of the normal father–mother influence. Stresses of various kinds and the slackening of old standards will endanger that atmosphere of security and harmony which are so necessary to satisfactory development.

Social welfare could not be neglected, particularly in respect of children.[22]

Manchester clinic staff had visited patients in the Reception Areas and the main problem was enuresis. 'In some cases', it was suggested, 'this is obviously a symptom which has been overlooked by the parents'. In others, though, 'it appears to be an anxiety response directly due to evacuation'. Two years later it was noted that while it was to be welcomed that the clinic was now dealing with a greater number of children of higher intelligence it was also true that 'it is the more intelligent who are liable to be disturbed and upset by the abnormality of their present lives' – a further instance of the perceived dangers to children of this sort. Clinic staff had participated in a survey of the effects of evacuation, the results of which had been published in *BMJ*.[23]

The Lanarkshire branch of the EIS, an organization actively involved in an area hosting many evacuees from Glasgow, prepared a report for the county's Education Committee on its experience. It was remarked that while it was not possible to establish statistically the need for a child guidance clinic it was unlikely that 'the situation in Lanarkshire, with the resulting need, differs materially' from those parts of Scotland and England where clinics had been founded. In organizational terms the experience of fully developed clinics was 'definitely in favour of a team of three – the psychiatrist, the clinical psychologist and the social worker with clerical assistance'. Child guidance was thus 'only partly a school medical service', having wider implications because of the 'psychological and sociological work it undertakes'. It was therefore concluded that child guidance was a state responsibility not least because voluntary clinics could not cope with the present situation. An increasing number of clinics were being established by local authorities with all 'available data and expert opinion' indicating the desirability of such institutions.[24] Once more we have a clear link between direct experience of evacuation and a demand for enhanced child guidance services. Unusually for Scotland psychiatry's role was also acknowledged.

But what of the more detailed investigations and analyses carried out in the wake of the first wave of evacuation and what they had to say about child guidance? The most famous of these surveys, that for Cambridge, is dealt with below in a section on wartime child guidance practice. In his contribution to the left-wing body the Fabian Society's survey, Bowlby first expressed a generally sympathetic view both of evacuees and their hosts noting that in peacetime the 'ill effects of bad homes have received far more attention than the good effects of the normal home'. He then remarked that those professionally involved with the 'psychological problems of family life' were 'surprised not at the breakdown of evacuation but at its partial success'. It was certainly the case that where possible small children should not be separated from their mothers. On the other hand, and especially in respect of older children the 'child who feels happy in his own home is the child who settles best in a foster-home. It is the child who has felt unhappy and insecure at home who finds it most difficult to leave it'.[25] These positions were not mutually contradictory: on the contrary they argued the centrality of the child's happiness within the family unit to its own and the family's future mental well-being. Evacuation as such was not, therefore, the problem. Rather what was important was to adopt, in the event of further possibilities of separation, psychologically sensitive policies which prioritized the quality of the child–parent relationship and its stage of development. This was a shift from Bowlby's earlier concerns about potentially widespread mental health problems to a position closer to that of Moodie's: that by and large evacuation exposed pre-existing problems. Equally, though, the case for services such as child guidance for the 'unhappy and insecure' is being made.

The report on Scotland was edited by the opponent of psychiatric child guidance, William Boyd, and none of its chapters were written by a medical doctor. Of particular interest was the contribution of Catherine McCallum, lead figure in the new, psychologically oriented local authority clinic opened in Glasgow in the late 1930s. McCallum noted that early reports from the Reception Areas suggested that a number of children were causing 'serious trouble' and that staff from Glasgow's psychological clinics had been sent to investigate. It was quickly realized that some of these children could not be billeted in the normal way and so the Nerston Residential Clinic, an 'Experiment in Child Guidance', was set up. All potential residents were screened for intelligence and 'mental defectives were refused'. Those who were simply unruly or badly controlled were likewise rejected and so all cases admitted were children with 'serious psychological problems'. Further evidence for admission certainly included 'reports of medical and psychiatric examinations'. But the Nerston team was led by a 'fully-qualified and experienced teacher-psychologist' supported by similarly trained staff. The institution was, McCallum suggested, 'first and foremost a home, then a school, then a clinic'. As to the children themselves:

> Little crippled personalities came there, hating, fearing, distrusting, their whole view of life distorted by their unhappiness. They leave again in six, twelve, or eighteen months, freer and happier individuals, grown whole again by self-knowledge, self-discipline, tolerance and sympathy for human weakness. It was upon these pillars that idealism raised the reality of Nerston.[26]

Here was an account which was unusual in child guidance in its resort to institutionalization but which shows too a self-confident and assertive view of psychologically driven theory and practice.

In the latter context it is worth noting the review, co-authored by Burt, of the Cambridge survey which had been carried out under the supervision of the eminent child psychologist, supporter of Melanie Klein and protégé of Burt's, Susan Isaacs. The review welcomed the survey as an important contribution to an understanding of children and their behaviour. It was also claimed that psychologists from other countries frequently enquired why in British child guidance

> the psychological characteristics of individual children are so commonly assessed by a physician rather than a psychologist fully trained in such work and why the physician does not report on the physical rather than on the mental condition of the children, especially when they are neither mentally diseased nor mentally defective.

Rather disingenuously the reviewers suggested that such enquires perhaps implied 'only a superficial knowledge of our methods'. But they also indicated 'where those who study our published reports feel that our scientific work is weak' - an implicit acknowledgement of the relatively undeveloped nature of psychology, at least in England. Further studies were called for and it was agreed that the assessment of child's health should be done by a doctor with specialist knowledge and not by anyone from any other profession. On the other hand, 'the psychological aspects of the study – the assessment of temperamental characteristics and the like – should be in the hands of a trained psychologist, not of a doctor, teacher, social worker, or psychiatrist'.[27] The review, in posing the question purportedly emanating from foreign psychologists, was clearly making the case for child guidance as a psychological rather than a medical service while linking it to the evacuation process.

Evacuation also affected child guidance in other ways. As with the Child Guidance Council, the LSE and the Diploma in Mental Health were moved to Cambridge. From the outset the School had been at pains to stress its commitment to the course with its Director writing to the Commonwealth Fund that it was of 'utmost importance' that it continue during the war. This was not least because, and reflecting the early wartime view that evacuation would of itself engender widespread mental health problems, '[t]housands of children have been evacuated from industrial areas, and personal problems in foster homes would seem inevitable'.[28]

From early 1941 students were also being trained in 'practical work in Child Guidance' in Oxford under the supervision of staff from the London Clinic directed by Fildes and financially underpinned by the Commonwealth Fund. This particular activity was later expanded to include the Abingdon Child Guidance Clinic.[29] Sybil Clement Brown, as well as working on the Cambridge Survey, also advised on that undertaken by social workers and psychologists from Barnett House in Oxford.[30] Brown in addition continued to proselytize for the LSE course. In a memorandum addressed to an American audience – almost certainly the Commonwealth Fund – around 1942, she stressed that one of its characteristics 'has been the close relationship maintained between the theoretical teaching and the practical experience'. Many of the course's staff had been trained in America and had 'tried to bring to the English course some of the quality of close interchange' between theory and practice they had found working in the US 'to such good effect'. Brown also noted the importance of support from Burt and the psychiatrists Moodie, Hart and Aubrey Lewis. She concluded that it was no longer necessary to convince students that in training to be PSWs they were 'undertaking something of national importance. This has become self-evident'.[31]

The Oxford region also saw a private initiative in child guidance. Early in 1940 the private Chelsea Open-Air Nursery School, which had been evacuated to

Oxfordshire, closed down. It then redeployed its resources to supply a psychiatrist, Miss E. V. Molteno, to provide diagnosis and treatment for all evacuee children. Hostels had been set up to house evacuees whose behaviour made them unfit for foster homes. In addition Molteno increasingly worked with local children, with schools and with the Oxford Child Guidance Clinic and had an input to the training for the LSE course. As the author of the article describing this development remarked, the 'number of difficult children appears to be unlimited'.[32]

Evacuation had initially been seen in child guidance circles as having the potential to further contribute to what was expected to be widespread psychological problems induced by war and, in particular, aerial bombardment. Such problems did not in any real sense materialize. Nonetheless, it was widely argued that evacuation had illuminated or brought into the open pre-existing instances of maladjustment. The evacuation experience also prompted new initiatives in child guidance practice, including institutions to deal with particularly disturbed children. And, itself evacuated, the LSE Mental Health course continued to train PSWs and to utilize to this end child guidance clinics outside London.

Evacuation in Britain also had an impact on thinking about child guidance overseas. In Australia an analysis was published at a time when that country was under threat of invasion and might thereby have needed to undertake evacuation. This publication remarked on the impact of emotional and behaviour problems on Britain's Reception Areas and, by the same token, the ability to call upon 'a considerable number of trained workers' from bodies such as child guidance clinics. For such workers emotional and behavioural problems 'were not evidence of "slum depravity" but the recognizable and curable reactions of children to difficult situations' – science displacing moralizing again. After an initial delay child guidance services had been variously expanded. Such clinics being virtually unknown in Australia, the lesson drawn was that in the event of evacuation 'child guidance clinics with staff of child psychiatrist, psychologist and social worker' should be established.[33] Two years later another author similarly noted child guidance's virtual absence in Australia and drew upon American and British experience to argue that his country's situation was 'not only unfair, even cruel, it is also extremely serious for society as a whole'. In Britain 'as a result of the extraordinary social conditions created by the war' there was being obtained 'new insights ... which will be of first importance to child guidance and the social sciences'. This author too supported the medical model.[34] The American Association of Psychiatric Social Workers, meanwhile, contacted its British counterpart seeking information 'on the whole question of the evacuation of the civilian population, children and adults' including what problems evacuees experienced and how they were treated.[35] For outside observers there was therefore a clear link between evacuation and child guidance.

Child Guidance Practice in Wartime

The ambiguity of the war in terms of its impact on child guidance was subsequently well brought out by the Underwood Committee. It was certainly the case that many promising pre-war developments came to a halt. Clinics lost staff and training was disrupted. On the other hand, and echoing other commentaries, evacuation had brought certain problems to light and, for the Reception Areas in particular, there was the bonus that child guidance practitioners not able to work in their home locations 'were spread throughout the country to help with the difficulties of children separated from their families'. It was through such experiences that 'the urgent need for child guidance and other facilities for the treatment of maladjusted children came to be recognised'.[36] We now turn to how child guidance operated in wartime with the focus, as previously, on its concern with maladjustment of the otherwise normal child.[37]

This is in the first instance illuminated by the most famous of the evacuation surveys, that of Cambridge. Collectively written under the supervision of Isaacs, contributors and participants included Bowlby, Sybil Clement Brown, LSE mental health students and PSWs loaned by the Mental Health Emergency Committee. The introduction noted that for successful billeting, 'experience in social work' and an 'understanding of the psychological needs of individual children' was invaluable and reinforced by 'the calls made upon the staff of the Child Guidance Training Centre'.[38] This argument was fleshed out in the chapter on 'Child Guidance in a Reception Area' on which the following discussion draws.

The situation in Cambridge in 1939 was that there was a part-time clinic operating out of the city's general hospital. Ten weeks into evacuation a training unit had been set up close to the hospital – almost certainly that noted above organized by the CGC – and, in cooperation with its child guidance clinic, offered practical training for seventeen LSE Mental Health course students. In practice the two locations acted as one combined training and clinical facility staffed by up to five psychiatrists, effectively two psychologists, a speech therapist and two full-time and one part-time social worker. The need for trained social workers was again stressed, not least because volunteers – much evacuation work was carried out by members of the Women's Voluntary Service (WVS) – were prone to misinterpret certain situations. This point was reiterated in a discussion of symptoms during which it was pointed out that some complaints against evacuees were unfounded or exaggerated.[39]

The child guidance approach when dealing with an evacuee population was carefully delineated. Evacuation had placed a considerable strain on some, but by no means all, children involved. Some had 'thriven happily on the new life in the country'. Others had however 'felt not only their own insecurity but that of their parents and homes'. In some cases children who had been difficult at home 'even

... in times of peace' had become worse while others had 'shown signs of strain for the first time'. In such circumstances, established child guidance techniques had to adapt to meet new challenges. Nonetheless, the aim in wartime and with evacuee children was the same as in peacetime with children in their own homes, namely to 'discover the child's capacity to meet the demands of life and to make such changes in his environment and in his personality as will help him to do so in the most constructive way'.[40] This was a revealing remark displaying a confidence in child guidance techniques far from universally shared.

As to the children themselves, 155 were treated over a ten-month period. Psychometric tests revealed IQ scores ranging from 59 to 151 with an average of 97 – as might by now be expected, these were for the most part 'normal' children. As in other clinics, boys predominated although here there was a huge disparity with boys constituting two-thirds of referrals. No particularly convincing explanation was given for this other than that boys might be more inclined to cause disturbances, especially in other people's homes. Because of the problems associated with voluntary workers the referral symptoms listed were interesting primarily 'in suggesting the difficulties most troublesome to local residents and to teachers rather than the true incidence of symptoms among children separated from their parents'. Bed-wetting, a very common cause of referral in peacetime and as noted a cause of resentment among those on whom children were billeted, topped this list with 48 per cent. Many of the remaining difficulties, it was suggested, 'are described by words which have no constant meaning, and the divisions between them may be arbitrary and relative to points of view about manners and morals'.[41] This suggests a confidence in scientific, professional child guidance techniques as opposed to the amateur, moralizing or simply prejudiced observations of WVS workers. Much of the backlash against evacuation derived from the reactions and reports of these predominantly middle-class women. But the survey's comments might also be seen as breathtakingly myopic given the clinical opacity of some child guidance terminology and the otherwise readily acknowledged problems of classification.

This last point is further illustrated by one of the survey's case studies of child guidance patients involving a 6-year old girl referred for bed-wetting and unexplained stomach pains. Her original foster home was of the 'superior' kind. It was at about the 'same social level as the child's own home' and the 'foster mother had sound principles of care and management'. Nonetheless the child, as well as displaying physical symptoms, was anxious and unhappy. She was then removed to a home 'run in a haphazard sort of way' where she became much more content. This haphazard home contained several generations, from babies to grandparents, and was characterized by 'much spontaneous affection'. Such an environment seemed to offer the kind of reassurance necessary to a child 'who had been distressed at home by scenes of violence between her two parents'.[42] It would be wrong to over-criticize such accounts and analyses not least because an unhappy child appears to have become happier. Nor do we have access to case notes, and clearly the child guidance workers were trying their best in extremely difficult and challenging circumstances. But it is difficult to see how describing a household as 'haphazard' or a foster mother as operating on sound principles of care and management differs, at least in a rhetorical sense, from the propensity to judge on the basis of morals and manners ascribed (undoubtedly correctly) to WVS members.

Other accounts further illuminate how child guidance operated in wartime. The Deputy Director of the Bristol clinic, Frank Bodman, reported to a wartime child guidance conference on a survey of 8,000 schoolchildren made in order to 'assess the incidence of strain following air raids'. Only 4 per cent showed any symptoms 'either purely psychological or else psycho-somatic'. He himself had examined a group which might have been expected to be especially traumatized. These were in-patients at the Children's Hospital when the latter was hit by high explosive bombs 'and the children were evacuated to another hospital at the height of the raid, under particularly trying circumstances'. Of the forty-four survivors, five still had symptoms attributable to that particular experience, all of them aged between one and five-and-a-half years. Nonetheless Bodman concluded, in line with other analyses, that the 'most striking result' of his survey was the 'extraordinary toughness of the child, and his flexibility in adapting to potentially threatening situations'.[43] Bristol clinic staff members more generally were, as a later report noted, 'devoted to problems arising directly and indirectly from the evacuation of the Bristol children' while the clinic itself suffered bomb damage and had to be relocated.[44]

In terms of the expansion of child guidance services, evacuation clearly provided impetus although it was also undoubtedly growing prior to 1939. As we have seen the APSW calculated that around the beginning of the war in England and Wales there were around fifty clinics of which just under half were wholly or partially maintained by local authorities. For Scotland the equivalent data were thirteen and just over one half.[45] The Underwood Committee recorded that by 1945 in England and Wales the number of clinics had risen to seventy-nine.[46] In Scotland data are harder to come by and because of the predominance of psychology, identifying what exactly constituted a child guidance clinic compounds the problem. But the Glasgow psychologist Catherine McCallum later recorded new clinics being founded in Fife and Edinburgh while educational psychologists were appointed by five local authorities.[47] This would suggest a total of around twenty.

For the most part, this expansion continued the pre-war trend of LEAs becoming more and more involved in actual provision. In Glasgow, for instance, the local authority not only set up the Nerston clinic in 1941; the following year 'war time experiences of disrupted education and juvenile delinquency' led to the decision to found 'three additional emergency clinics', thereby setting up a system of child guidance which was to last in the city for the next two decades.[48] In Edinburgh, meanwhile, and bearing out McCallum's point, the *Scotsman* reported that it had been agreed by the local authority that it would be 'desirable to establish a child guidance scheme that would deal with the problem of maladjusted children systematically and comprehensively'. In Scottish fashion the first step was deemed to be the appointment of a psychologist whose initial task would be to survey existing provision and the situation in general.[49] The Commonwealth Fund noted in 1944 that some county councils were now taking an interest in child guidance and thereby spreading the work 'out into rural neighbourhoods'.[50]

Despite growing local authority involvement, voluntarism had far from disappeared. In July 1942 it was agreed to set up a Child Guidance Council for Northern Ireland. The consequent clinic, the first of its kind in Ireland as a whole, was to be connected with Belfast's Hospital for Sick Children. Funding had come in the form of £1,000 from an anonymous donor and £2,000 given by the Queen from the 'Bundles for Britain Fund'.[51] At Notre Dame in Glasgow an annual grant of £650 from the local authority was certainly a key element of financial support. But a 1945 memorandum also noted the continuing support of the Notre Dame Convent in terms of accommodation and its upkeep, voluntary labour on the part of community members and the 'many charitable friends and institutions' such as the St Vincent de Paul Society.[52] Voluntary labour of another kind could be found at various centres. In Birmingham, Burns successfully lobbied councillors to allow for the employment on an unpaid basis of a Dr Spies from Worms and a Dr Elner from Vienna, refugee doctors from Nazi-occupied Europe.[53] The East London Jewish Clinic also had refugee social workers and doctors on its staff prior to the outbreak of war and given government restrictions the latter at least were almost certainly unpaid.[54]

Of course by the 1940s the level of Commonwealth Fund support had dramatically reduced despite efforts by the LSE and CGC to have it maintained. Indeed, Fund officials frequently complained about the behaviour of LSE officials, which had been a concern from the beginning. One internal document remarked that promoting mental hygiene in England had involved dealing with 'some very astute and not always completely ingenuous people' and so had been challenging, interesting and exasperating. Another document noted Scoville's visit in 1939 and that she was taking a tough line in her negotiations, something which had the personal approval of Edward Harkness. The same document commented that getting those in Britain to take responsibility for child guidance and PSW training had been the 'hardest nut to crack in the Fund's experience'. This was in part due to British ineptitude at raising philanthropic support and a perceived attitude that the Fund would always come to the rescue.[55] In any event Fund support, which had peaked in 1933/4 at nearly $87,000, by 1945 was down to under $19,000.[56]

So the CGC in particular had to look elsewhere for financial resources and in 1944 received a grant of £4,500 from the British philanthropic body the Nuffield Foundation. This was 'mainly used for training purposes a special sum having been set aside for the training of psychiatrists returning from the services'.[57] Important as this was, the wider context is revealing about the rest of the voluntary mental health movement's attitude to child guidance, purportedly one of its most important components. At the beginning of 1944 St Loe Strachey wrote to Janet Vaughan at the Nuffield that it was 'unfortunately quite true that what we need is an immediate grant'. The other constituent parts of the Provisional National Council for Mental Health did not, she continued, 'see that Child Guidance is of urgent importance as the foundation of the whole Mental Health Movement', the broader situation here being the imminent formation of the National Association for Mental Health (NAMH). These other parts were inclined to think that 'any haphazard arrangements will do for Clinics' and when after the war amalgamation eventually came about, unless the CGC was 'a going concern and financially sound and solvent, an insufficient grant will be allotted to it'. In turn, this would undermine 'the high standard of work which is necessary in the National interest'. A subsequent letter, noting the demise of Commonwealth Fund support, asked for £3,000 per annum and suggested that this would be used for training child psychiatrists and psychologists and for organizational purposes.[58] The larger but one-off grant resulted. And to illustrate further the problems of fundraising, the NAMH recorded in 1947 that a bid for £12,000 per annum from the Nuffield to support the training of psychiatrists, psychologists, PSWs and non-medical therapists 'sufficient to meet about half the requirements anticipated in the next ten years' for child guidance had been turned down.[59] Voluntarism thus still had a role to play in child guidance during the war and was to continue to do so through the NAMH. Voluntary funding was, though, a problematic issue.

After the War is Over

So far we have seen how child guidance anticipated and responded to evacuation and its consequences and the practical implications for service provision amid the disruptions of war. We now examine how, while the conflict was still going on, some of its leading proponents envisaged child guidance in the post-war world. This is less to do with the active campaigns to pressurize government, dealt with in the next chapter, and more about the intellectual underpinnings and intellectual differences over the direction in which child guidance should travel. The starting point is a speech by Miller at a conference organized by the CGC in 1941, the event at which Bodman had reported on the results of his Bristol survey.

Miller was primarily concerned with the future but he did begin with an analysis of evacuation which, he agreed, had certainly been a huge upheaval. But it had also enabled the study of 'social and psychological phenomena as they have never been studied before' and from such studies 'we will draw wisdom for a future mental hygiene plan'. Evacuees thus had to be 'studied scientifically – for the data to be revealed will be of practical value'. Like Bowlby, Miller separated out the experience of evacuation, which clearly had negative aspects, from its more positive lessons. Once the war was over, Miller continued, it would be necessary to convince government that the 'care of the minds of the children is the best insurance against future wars, and the best safeguard against any form of social decay or upheaval'. This would require state intervention, as for too long child guidance had been dependent on 'the good will of private enthusiasm, wealth and enterprise'. State financial investment was required to ensure the mental well-being of children and, thereby, the broader society – an essentially prophylactic approach. So in each locality mechanisms should be set up whereby the 'trinity of physical health, mental health and social relations' could be studied, since not enough account was taken of the 'social anthropology of our contemporary society'. It was necessary to study group behaviour for 'mental hygiene must evolve from a given society – it cannot by imposed by a professional board dictating from a remote academic seat of omniscience'. As one speaker remarked in the ensuing discussion, Miller was asking, in effect, for a 'new social philosophy'.[60]

Miller's proposals at their most prosaic involved systematic state funding of child guidance. At their most visionary, child guidance was to be part of a wider mission to utilize all intellectual resources available, and new organizational forms, to bring about and maintain the future mental health of both children and society as a whole. Clearly this was an ambitious project for the post-war world and some of the problems in realizing it were to emerge at the other wartime conference we discuss here and which took place two years later. Held under the auspices of the Provisional National Council for Mental Health this was the sixth Child Guidance Interclinic Conference. The opening address was given by Burns and was important both in the issues it raised and the discussion and disagreement it provoked.

Burns's first major point conceded that there remained a certain imprecision as to the subject of their endeavours, quite correctly as 'child guidance is by no means a static thing; it is always changing its concepts and its own idea of itself'. Nonetheless, the work undertaken was 'absorbing, fruitful and immensely worthwhile', if not always subject to quantitative assessment. All this was uncontroversial enough in that there were acknowledged definitional problems in assessing the success of child guidance and even its area of concern. But then Burns moved, probably deliberately, into more contentious areas. It was necessary to end the 'unreal, fruitless and pernicious academic discussion' which had been aired in certain quarters as to whether 'clinics should be medical or psychological, whether they should be called "clinics" or "centres" and whether the children are sick or normal with deviations'. Rather, it should be recognized that 'child guidance' in the broad sense was 'practically synonymous with the mental health of childhood'. As such it embraced the psychological dimensions of the School Medical Service which should in fact be doing much of the work presently done in clinics. The latter could be run in various ways, but whatever the organizational form, 'the psychiatric side must never be neglected'. Even though not in charge, the child psychiatrist must be 'an integral partner in the work and not just somebody called in for the odd consultation'. As to what psychiatrists actually did, Burns argued that they should, 'generally speaking, see only those cases in which psychiatry really comes into question and should have far more time and opportunity for therapy'. Psychologists and PSWs could thus be given more responsibility for handling cases not needing direct psychiatric intervention.[61]

This was not an entirely coherent argument – the case for a continuing centrality, even predominance, of psychiatry, for instance, was rather at odds with condemnation of purportedly sterile academic debates. Burns's speech did nonetheless raise important issues, some of which had been present more or less from the beginning. Others were developmental in the sense that, as Burns noted, what actually constituted child guidance was fluid and subject to change. The broader context is also important. As arguments for greater child guidance provision intensified, so greater definitional clarity was sought, an issue we return to in the next chapter. But for present purposes we might note two further aspects of the speech. First, we have the recognition of a division over the medical versus psychological approach. Burns sought to dismiss such a division but it was fundamental – it really did matter whether children were seen as 'sick' or 'normal with deviations' and this was not going to be brushed under the carpet. Second, there was the question of what the child guidance psychiatrist should actually do. For Burns fewer cases and more intensive therapy was the answer, a reflection of his own growing personal and professional interests.

His approach was shared by others. Dr Edelston of the Bradford Clinic thought it important that clinics never 'degenerate into an intensive social service at the cost of the deep therapy'. One implication of this was that the psychiatrist must be the 'diagnostician of the clinic'. This was not least because in deciding which child patients should receive deep therapy, which only psychiatrists could do, he or she was also making a judgement about all those to whom deep therapy was not applicable. Edelston also made far-reaching and rather emotive claims for the mission of child guidance, going even further than Miller's 'new social philosophy'. Whether or not child guidance workers realized it, one consequence of their treatment of children was that 'they were preaching a moral for the handling of all children' – a logical enough point and one to which most child guidance practitioners would have subscribed given the didactic dimension of their work. Edelston took this further, though, suggesting that one implication of this role was that he and his co-workers were 'revolutionaries of the first order, and that was why they had so much trouble'. They were 'preaching personal freedom' and this was something which practitioners had to confront.[62] This is almost certainly a reflection of the times – an era of intense debate about post-war social reconstruction – rather than a serious proposal about child guidance's future role. But it is rather different from Moodie's assertion of the need for a balance between freedom and discipline something which as we shall see was to be reformulated as the welfare state was being constructed.

Others took a different view of Burns's speech, notably MacCalman. He summed up the former's address as essentially arguing that 'psychiatrists must have more real cases, ie. they must have a higher percentage of cases which required intensive therapy'. Another approach, though, was that psychiatrists should 'almost neglect cases that were really ill in favour of treating cases which were fundamentally normal but were in temporary difficulty'. Such a strategy, which had been adopted in the armed services, would be unpopular with both the general public and the Treasury. The former would see the most difficult cases in the community not being immediately treated while the latter would resist such an approach 'because it was a long term one'. Nonetheless child guidance professionals must 'avoid being overburdened by clinical material of a very acute kind and turn to the real work of prevention and planning for positive mental health'.[63] Burns, summing up the morning session, stressed that he had not intended to belittle psychiatric work in, for instance, the 'preventive and the educational fields'. Nonetheless, he agreed with a speaker who had suggested that the child guidance clinic should be the apex of the child guidance pyramid and that clinics' work should thereby be 'intensified and made more therapeutic'.[64]

The conference's afternoon session was particularly focused more on the issue of treatment and so, inevitably, the psychiatrists' role came up again. In a rare intervention in such debates, Donald Winnicott noted the 'tremendous demand which existed for actual therapy of individual children' in tandem with the danger of 'child guidance workers forgetting how little they knew' – something of a slight to his professional colleagues although, on the other hand, something which the more open of them acknowledged. To those who thought that play therapy was all that was required, he responded that it was of use only when children were 'normal'. He himself was not ashamed to be 'associated with psychoanalysts who did not consider it was a bad thing to treat one child every day for a year or two'. This was almost certainly a reference to the work of Klein with whom Winnicott was at this point associated.[65]

Conclusion

More fault lines appear, alerting us once more to important divisions within British child guidance. Winnicott's use of the word 'normal' is somewhat ambiguous although not entirely incompatible with mainstream child guidance psychiatric discourse. His rather patronizing criticism of play therapy, though, was controversial, at least to this particular audience, as was his forthright advocacy of psychoanalysis. In turn this leads to more general and fundamental questions concerning the role in child guidance for both psychiatry and the clinic. Was the latter, for instance, in the front line of preventive medicine and mental health promotion among children, as MacCalman suggested? Such an approach, in association with the centrality of the 'normal' child, had been foundational to British child guidance. Or was it a specialized, therapeutic and intensive unit at the apex of a broader mental health programme, with the latter seeking to promote child guidance in a much more encompassing way wherein it was even prepared to cede clinical ground to psychologists and PSWs? If so, did this indicate that some psychiatrists were moving away from the environmental approach to engage with one emerging trend in what was increasingly being called child psychiatry, the trend sympathetic to psychoanalysis? Child guidance thus remained full of tensions and these continued to play themselves out in the post-war era. Nonetheless, as we shall see in the next chapter, as plans for social reconstruction developed during the early 1940s proponents of child guidance, unofficial and official, successfully pressed the case for increased provision, with child guidance becoming part of the emerging welfare state.

6 CHILD GUIDANCE AND THE BRITISH WELFARE STATE

Introduction

In this chapter we first analyse the claims for enhanced child guidance provision from both outside and inside central government. Partly as a result of the evacuation experience, although also in line with pre-war trends, child guidance proponents argued that maladjustment was a national problem which had to be dealt with nationally. Such arguments were successful in that by way of the Education Acts of the mid-1940s, child guidance was legislatively embedded in the emerging welfare state. It is thus crucial to see child guidance as part of, and contributing to, a broad wave of social reconstruction which began to take shape in Britain as the war came to an end. Child guidance took its place alongside such new services as socialized health care and state-provided family allowances in the attempt by the British state to protect its citizens against unforeseen problems and to promote social stability, social solidarity and social harmony. Such aims were broadly agreed and came to be seen as a key constituent of Britain's political and social post-war consensus. In this context we also examine what it was that child guidance's advocates saw it as contributing to social reconstruction and the extent of child guidance services by the mid-1950s. Legislation and expansion notwithstanding, child guidance remained a contested field and we shall see how Scottish provision came to influence that elsewhere in Britain.

Promoting Child Guidance: Outside Central Government

As evidence of the impact of evacuation accumulated, as plans for post-war reconstruction were increasingly discussed and as more child guidance clinics opened, the child guidance message continued to be promoted in various ways. The period 1942–3 – when plans for and debates over post-war reconstruction were in full flow – was particularly crucial. Interventions ranged from public talks by practitioners through specific demands emanating from voluntary organizations, professional bodies and local authorities. To these we should add the voices heard in previous chapters from interested parties such as the Scottish

Women's Group on Public Welfare and the contributions of leading child guidance practitioners to professional meetings in 1941 and 1943.

Dr Grace Calver, psychiatrist at the Tavistock and at the Maidenhead Child Guidance Clinic, was part of a programme funded by the Central Council for Health Education under the general rubric 'Rural Mental Health Education'. Her lecture series, delivered to bodies such as women's institutes, was entitled 'Understanding Ourselves and Our Children'. Calver, describing her activities, claimed to have gone to considerable pains to avoid jargon and phrases such as 'child complexes' and was thus utilizing the previously encountered popularizing and didactic approach. She compared emotional development to physical development, something which most parents could understand, with the broad aim of promoting 'emotional health'. Most physical ailments, Calver claimed, resulted from 'emotional conflicts and disharmonies which upset the normal bodily functions' and hence 'emotional and mental health' was fundamental to all preventive medicine. There was obviously a great need for clinics to which problems could be referred but the present dearth of such institutions was 'no argument against giving Mental Health lectures'. To illustrate the point she gave the example of a mother's changed attitude to a 3-year-old child caught lying, when it was pointed out to the former that 'a child that age looks at the world in an entirely different light, and its interpretation of a happening may be wrong'.[1] Calver was thus bringing her professional insights to a much wider audience. This audience was based in the countryside where child guidance had as yet made few inroads. She also made clear the need for more clinics while emphasizing an idea often left implicit in child guidance, that emotional health was important to physical well-being.

A Child Guidance Council member told the 1943 meeting of the National Conference on Maternity and Child Welfare that the family was 'the essential basic relationship' in childrearing. Nevertheless 'we seemed to think that the very getting together of a family was of itself a panacea which needed no science and which needed no social training behind it'. The experience of child guidance now suggested that this was not so. The 'very fact' of motherhood 'did not necessarily make one the best person for bringing up one's child without further education and elucidation of the problems concerned'. Here we once more encounter an emphasis on professional intervention on a scientific basis alongside potential maternal inadequacies. Consequently, Miss Thomas continued, the Council was 'turning its views more and more to the realisation of the importance of preventive work in the field of health', not least because therapeutic knowledge was 'not yet profound enough to make us able to do many of the things we would want to do with the 1 per cent of sick children who needed our help'. And in administrative terms it was unlikely that sufficient psychological help would be universally available within the next twenty or thirty years. So the prevention of 'such a state of inner turmoil and tension' in order to head off abnormality and difficulty was 'one of the big problems' on which the Council was increasingly focusing its attention.[2] Parental education as a key constituent of a preventive mental health programme, in other words, was a central child guidance concern.

Cyril Burt reported to the BPS Council in 1944 that the transmission of the Society's views to central government on the current Education Bill, gathered by his Committee on Reconstruction and 'which was the most urgent of the Committee's tasks, was now completed'. In consequence, the Committee was wound up. While not specifically mentioning child guidance it seems highly improbable, given developments within the BPS discussed in the next chapter, that Burt would have omitted this from his suggestions to the Board.[3]

The message being put forward by practitioners and activists was also pressed by lay bodies. The Standing Joint Committee of Working Women's Organizations, active in the 1930s in promoting child guidance, wrote to the Board of Education in late 1941 to impress on it 'the need for the provision by local authorities of Child Guidance Clinics'. Many Committee members had social work experience, especially with children's courts, and were of the view that 'wartime conditions' had made the provision of child guidance 'more urgent than ever'.[4] Such interventions illustrate the political weight accorded to post-war reconstruction in the early 1940s. In 1943, meanwhile, the National Union of Women Teachers wrote to MPs to alert them to resolutions passed at its annual conference, including that 'Child Guidance clinics should be provided'.[5]

Later the same year Leah Manning, one of the leaders of the National Union of Teachers and future Labour MP, suggested in *Mother and Child* that among the essentials for child care in any National Health Service – a topic much discussed especially since the recent publication of the Beveridge Report – would be child guidance clinics.[6] Also in 1943, the LCC noted that, its longstanding support for child guidance notwithstanding, up to that point its policy had 'been marked by caution'. However, the Council had recently investigated the provision of twenty-one other local education authorities and concluded that there 'appears to be a growing desire to make provision for dealing with the maladjusted child and the general opinion is that the work should be in close association with, if not an integral part of, the school medical service'.[7] From a variety of standpoints, then, the child guidance message continued to be vigorously promoted by organizations and individuals outside of central government.

Promoting Child Guidance: Inside Central Government

As we have seen, the Board of Education had paid close attention to child guidance from the outset and had in the mid-1930s taken policy initiatives which had enabled local authorities to found or support clinics. The relatively positive attitude of the Board, now under the supervision of Churchill's coalition government, was strengthened by the wartime experience. In 1941 arguments were put forward by civil servants for legislation to at the very least encourage greater child guidance provision. It was noted that medical treatment for school children varied among local authorities, with some providing only the bare minimum but others including services such as 'the treatment of maladjusted children through child guidance clinics or otherwise'. Such differences were partly due to the very nature of local government provision but also reflected a lack of definition as to what constituted medical care. Persuasion, it was suggested, did not usually work so there was a need for legislation to secure all of the services indicated and including child guidance.[8] The issue of evacuees and child guidance also exercised the official mind. A Board memorandum from 1942 remarked that 'several schemes for child guidance treatment are being or have been considered jointly by ourselves and the Ministry of Health'. The particular focus here was on Buckinghamshire and Berkshire where it was noted that services were required to deal with both 'native' and evacuated children.[9]

In the same year the Board responded to a Ministry of Health query regarding the value of the latter continuing a grant to the Mental Health Emergency Committee. At the heart of this was the training of PSWs. Acknowledging various problems associated with this scheme, the Board nonetheless suggested that the grant continue. There had been, it noted, a small increase in child guidance provision during the preceding year. Although rapid expansion was out of the question because of overall staff shortages, nonetheless 'we should like to see further Training Courses provided in order to supply the most essential part of the staff of any Child Guidance arrangements, namely, the PSWs'. It was further the case that while psychologists were fairly hard to find, 'they do exist'. Psychiatrists, on the other hand, were 'more or less unobtainable' although School Medical Officers could to some degree fulfil this role. But aside from the continuing financial support, what is revealing about this correspondence is the centrality in the Board's eyes of the PSW. This point was reiterated in the document's conclusion which suggested that the 'sine qua non of any [child guidance] scheme is ... the trained PSW and there can be virtually no further development of schemes unless the supply of these is increased'.[10] What is implicit here is that child guidance provision should be expanded, although given the centrality of the social worker's role it could be legitimately argued that the Board's attitude suggested that it was to be seen as a sort of social service within the existing educational and school medical structures and certainly not one dominated by psychiatry.

Support for child guidance could be found at the Board's highest level. Its president, the Conservative minister R. A. Butler, recorded a meeting with a Home Office civil servant in late 1942. The Home Office was responsible for areas of welfare and justice contiguous with or even overlapping child guidance. The official thus argued that his department was 'determined not to alter the arrangements for delinquent and mal-adjusted children'. In response Butler pointed out that the 'psychological treatment of delinquent and mal-adjusted children had greatly developed, and Child Guidance Clinics were run by the LEAs'. Pressing his point home, he 'indicated the number and nature of the educational bodies' which had approached the Board 'with a view to encouraging the organisation of the care of these children by the Board of Education'.[11] Again this is about more than civil service territorial struggles – the clear implication is that child guidance provision should be increased and that the Board was the body which should be in overall control of this process. Butler himself took an interest in mental health issues. After the war he became president of the NAMH, the campaigning body into which the CGC had been merged, and was chair of the first conference of the World Federation of Mental Health in London in 1948. Child guidance activists such as Priscilla Norman, moreover, clearly found him a sympathetic character.[12]

Child guidance thus featured, if only fleetingly, in proposals for educational reconstruction put to the War Cabinet in summer 1943. In the section on 'Medical Inspection and Treatment' it was again noted that practices varied widely between local authorities. Citing earlier Board documents, it was further observed that some LEAs provided just the bare minimum while others, albeit only a few, had services including 'the treatment of maladjusted children through child guidance clinics or otherwise'. The clear drift of the argument was that the more comprehensive model was to be aspired to and that local authorities have the 'duty' placed upon them to deliver both medical inspection and treatment to any child who needed it.[13] While hardly a major foregrounding of child guidance, its presence as part of educational reconstruction nonetheless suggests that it was by now seen as an integral part of any future school medical service, a reasonable achievement given that it had been generally unheard of two decades previously.

This is not to say that child guidance supporters and practitioners felt sure of its proper acknowledgement in government circles and their own place in social reconstruction. In 1944 the Provisional National Council for Mental Health suggested that in 'plans for reconstruction, whatever form of Mental Health Committee is suggested for an area, voluntary associations should form part and there should be a national body to coordinate information and action'.[14] To put it another way, voluntarism should continue to have a role in any expanded child guidance services and the latter should not, thereby, simply be the responsibility of the state. Given the medical model of child guidance to which this body adhered, its argument might also suggest concerns over the way child guidance was being embraced by the welfare state.

Two years earlier the psychiatrist R. G. Gordon, on behalf of the CGC and the Mental Health Emergency Committee, wrote to Butler expressing concern that in the latter's recent statements on educational reconstruction 'little or no attention has been drawn to the promotion and preservation of the Mental Health of Children'. It had been the Council's experience in its fourteen years of existence that 'it had the sympathy and helpful cooperation of your Department'. It was therefore to be hoped that in future education plans 'the Mental Health and Happiness and emotional stability of children will not be lost sight of, especially as the neglect of this aspect of Child Health so often interferes with the full fruits of education'.[15] Butler sought to reassure Gordon. The 'development of child guidance work through clinics and in other ways', he claimed, 'will be fully considered as part of the plans for post-war educational reform'. The Board also valued 'the work done by the Child Guidance Council to promote and preserve the mental health of children'.[16] While as we have seen Butler seems to have been predisposed to sympathy for child guidance, positive interventions by his own officials and by professionals such as Gordon may have helped him clarify his own ideas and consolidate child guidance in the plans for educational reconstruction.

In Scotland Tom Johnston, the Secretary of State and active proponent of post-war reconstruction, was concerned about a perceived increase in juvenile delinquency. This resulted in a national convention on the subject and subsequently an official committee to enquire into the treatment and rehabilitation of offenders. One member of the committee, whose deliberations ranged more widely than juvenile delinquency as such, was Sister Marie Hilda and evidence was heard from a number of those directly or indirectly involved with child guidance. D. K. Henderson, for example, recommended more 'well-equipped Child Guidance Clinics'. MacCalman, meanwhile, argued for a broadly based approach which included, but did not exclusively rely upon, child guidance – a more encompassing mental health strategy was required. At the same meeting MacCalman suggested that Scotland was a 'matriarchal society' in the sense that it was the mother who had 'the greatest influence in the upbringing of the children'.[17] Such a belief could, of course, be used to justify an approach which in principle targeted all parents for education in childrearing but in fact tended to focus on the mother.

Scotland and Psychology Revisited

The nature of Scottish child guidance also had particular policy ramifications. In spring 1943 Dr A. F. Alford of the School Medical Service and one of His Majesty's Inspectors of Education, Mr J. Lumsden, visited Scotland on behalf of the Board of Education.[18] The trip's origins lay in recent contacts with the CGC, child guidance clinics and some LEAs. These discussions had uncovered 'marked differences of opinion ... upon the directions in which expansion should take place'. These differences involved matters of administration, the relationship with other health and education services and which types of staff should be employed. There had been criticism of 'what might be called the orthodox view expressed by the Child Guidance Council' and this criticism had in some cases been 'buttressed by examples taken from Scottish practice'.

In the course of their visit Alford and Lumsden met with various Scottish practitioners, including Drever. The latter, while claiming to have specifically medical input to his clinic, nonetheless argued that psychology was a science distinct from and independent of medicine. Unsurprisingly, he rejected the idea that psychologists should have no clinical role in child guidance. The visitors seemed persuaded by this sort of claim while noting that doctors in Scotland were prepared to work more collaboratively with other clinic staff than in England and did not seek to dominate the field. Consequently child guidance was viewed as more an educational than a medical issue and indeed the only Scottish clinic which followed the 'American methods of the Child Guidance Council' was Notre Dame (which was led, as Alford and Lumsden also remarked, by the trained psychologist Sister Marie Hilda).

Summing up, Alford and Lumsden observed that what 'we saw in Scotland clarified and reinforced the views which we had already formed from our experience [in England]', namely that if child guidance was 'to develop in the best way it must be regarded as an aspect of education rather than as an aspect of health'. There was a danger that plans now being formulated for widespread adult mental health services might include services such as child guidance, thereby 'linking it with the mental hospitals and outpatient clinics rather than with education. We believe this to be wrong in principle'. The Board should thus resist any attempt to make child guidance the sole responsibility of any health authority. The two argued instead that 'the linking of the maladjusted child with other types of handicapped children should be recognised, thus emphasising the educational aspect of child guidance' – more or less exactly what transpired. One consequence of this was that if psychiatrists were to be involved they should not be, as was the case in England at present, separate from the School Medical Service. The Scottish practice of having psychologists trained as teachers, moreover, clearly caught their attention and favour. The officials' report also emphasized the centrality of the PSW, as had other Board documents, and that child guidance should be concerned with educating parents and teachers as well as dealing directly with troubled children.

In policy context Wooldridge points to the influence of psychologists on plans for educational reconstruction notwithstanding their more general disciplinary weakness and the opportunity afforded, and taken, by the 1944 Act for the expansion of educational psychology and its employment in child guidance clinics.[19] And as Thom observes, the war put 'educational psychologists on the map' and 'accentuated their claim to a permanent place in the education system as mediators between society and the educators'.[20]

Psychology's contemporary aspirations regarding child guidance are clearly illustrated by Burt's arguments in the 1944 edition of his influential work *The Young Delinquent*. In a section specifically devoted to child guidance clinics he pointed to recent refutations of the idea that misbehaviour was a form of mental illness, to the acknowledged weakness of psychiatric training and to psychiatrists' lack of experience with children and their problems – by now familiar claims. Burt further pointed to divergences of opinion within psychiatry and in particular between psychoanalysts and those who saw mental illness as fundamentally caused by organic problems. In a rather curious leap of logic he then remarked that 'psychologists, on the other hand, maintain that psychology, by its very definition, takes the entire human personality as its province'. Except for pathological cases, especially rare in children, delinquency was therefore 'a natural and normal reaction to social situations that are in themselves more or less abnormal or unnatural'. Psychologists thus maintained that 'psychological and social measures are of the first importance, and medical, surgical, and psychiatrical [*sic*] of only occasional or incidental value'. And where clinics reported successes this could be as much due to staff taking a sympathetic approach to parents and their children as to diagnoses which stressed, possibly mistakenly, underlying pathology. The psychologist's or doctor's personality therefore had much to do with effecting 'cures'. Burt thus argued for a comprehensive and eclectic approach, something which he felt had in fact been increasingly occurring in recent years.[21] His own scepticism about psychiatry and psychiatrically based child guidance nonetheless was all too evident and by now widely shared.

Embedding Child Guidance in the Welfare State

But to return to the actual policy process, the end result of pre-war innovations and wartime experience, discussion and proselytizing was that child guidance was legislatively embedded in the emerging welfare state through the Education Act 1944 and the Education (Scotland) Act 1945. These Acts were less politically contentious, even consensual, parts of the emerging welfare state. The Scottish Act explicitly used the term 'child guidance' although maladjustment as a category was eschewed in favour of 'handicapped, backward, and difficult children'.[22] During its Second Reading the Scottish Secretary, Johnston, suggested that his recent conference on delinquency had clearly demonstrated child guidance to be a 'service of primary importance'.[23]

The 1944 Act, though, does not explicitly mention either 'child guidance' or 'maladjustment', although of course in general terms what it did was to expand and consolidate the function of LEA school medical services.[24] But it is clear from other documentary sources, including some of those discussed earlier in this chapter, both what was intended and what was involved. So, for instance, the Board of Education told the Board of Control in spring 1944 that logically there was

> of course a good case for the Child Guidance service, insofar as it deals with deep rooted maladjustments, neurosis and psychosis in children, being the responsibility of the Authority which deals with mental aberration among the adult population ... Logic, however, may carry us away from realities.

For one thing and echoing Burt, the number of children who presented deep-rooted abnormalities at clinics was small and in any event, if child guidance was to achieve anything, it had to be closely associated with schools. There were, too, objections to associating child guidance with mental hospitals. So child guidance clinics should come under the LEA remit. The SMO should be in charge although clinics should also be able to call on the services of a psychiatrist.[25] As we shall see presently, SMOs had their own views of how the new service should be run and some at least were much more sympathetic to their fellow doctors, the psychiatrists, than might have been anticipated.

The CMO to the Ministry of Education (the Board's successor) likewise had no doubts on the matter in the report on wartime education. As far as he was concerned LEAs now had the 'statutory duty to provide adequate and efficient arrangements, not only for the ascertainment of maladjusted children but also for their special educational treatment'. While most could be dealt with in school by educational psychologists there were also many who required 'treatment' because their 'maladjustments have some underlying emotional or personality factors which cause the deviation from the normal'. Such cases should be referred to child guidance clinics under the 'clinical charge of a psychiatrist'.[26] The Underwood Committee in 1955 too suggested that the 1944 Act had provided 'further impetus to the treatment of maladjusted children'. This had been consolidated by the Handicapped Pupils and School Health Service Regulations of 1945 which had included, for the first time, 'maladjustment' as falling within the definition of 'handicapped'.[27] The grounds for this had been laid by, for example, a memorandum from Butler to the War Cabinet Legislation Committee in late 1943 which had noted that 'the duty of ascertainment of defective children is extended to include all children needing special educational treatment'.[28] In short, child guidance was to be primarily a function of the School Medical Service. Particularly in the Scottish case this is unsurprising. It was not, though, uncontested outside Scotland. Given that child guidance's medical proponents had often been at pains to assert their authority over psychologists and educational psychologists, the relationship with the School Medical Service was not a development entirely to be welcomed.

A memorandum on 'Psychiatrists in the Child Guidance Services' was sent to the Board of Education by the Council of the Royal Medico-Psychological

Association in late 1944. This argued that irrespective of how child guidance clinics were administered, and on whose behalf, 'treatment should be under the direction of the psychiatrist'. The Council also claimed that 'every clinic should have available the services of a psychiatrist for purposes, not only of treatment, but also of diagnosis' [emphases in the original]. It was recognized that the rapid expansion of child guidance clinics had raised supply problems in respect of appropriately trained psychiatrists and this was something which the Council itself had to address. It also recognized and regretted that

> with the development of the Child Guidance movement, friction has here and there occurred between the claims of psychologists and psychiatrists. The Council holds that the Child Guidance services of the future will develop most harmoniously and efficiently if psychologists, psychiatric social workers and psychiatrists be encouraged to regard one another as colleagues, working in a team.

Nonetheless, and unremittingly, medicine's leading role was emphasized.[29]

Similarly, the APSW at the end of a discussion of the 1944 NHS White Paper agreed that a psychiatrist should be in charge of 'the treatment clinic' and that this should be part of a comprehensive health service. This, it was felt, would help ensure 'our decision at an earlier meeting that the family should be treated as a unit'. In the event of an educational psychologist being in charge of a clinic run by an LEA 'we would hope to see her [*sic*] used in co-operation with the health service'.[30]

School Medical Officers too had strong views on the control of any new service. In the mid-1940s the Association of Education Committees suggested that the staffing of a child guidance service in larger areas should consist of the usual personnel, including a psychiatrist capable of both diagnosis and treatment. But this team should also contain an educational psychologist, equally capable of diagnosis and treatment. In small areas only a part-time psychiatrist would be required with the strong implication thereby that the educational psychologist would take the lead.[31] SMOs reacted strongly to this claim. Any child guidance service, it was argued, should be under the control of the SMO. With regard to treatment it was strongly felt that this 'must be under the supervision of the Medical Psychiatrist'. The latter might delegate certain tasks, but it had to be stressed that overall the majority of child guidance cases were 'medico-psychological' rather than 'educational'. Hence it would be 'as ill-advised to entrust this work to an Educational Psychologist as it would be to entrust an orthopaedic scheme to a Physical Training Inspector'.[32] This was hardly a flattering comment and further explains the resentment many psychologists felt to their medically trained colleagues. But it also illustrates professional solidarity among doctors even from those who might be thought to have had their own territorial claims in the expanding School Medical Service.

Here it is also worth noting a delegation of SMOs to the Ministry of Education in 1948, which does not appear to have been a happy occasion. It was observed that the Permanent Secretary had suggested that any LEA should, in respect of child guidance, 'be entirely free to do what it liked'. Dr Alford, one of the wartime delegation to Scotland, then made the 'catastrophic remark' to the effect that most child guidance work was chiefly educational. To this Dr Alfred Newth, whom we shall encounter in the next chapter as Senior SMO for Nottingham, 'replied most emphatically no'.[33]

But all this was something of a losing battle and here, first, we should recognize the limitations of, and limits to, social reconstruction and not least the staffing problems in child guidance. In 1942, even as plans for post-war social reform were taking off, the APSW was reminded by a doctor from the CGC that 'the present shortage of psychiatrists for Child Guidance Work was likely to continue after the war'. It was thus recommended that individuals qualified as PSWs or educational psychologists 'could be given additional training' enabling them to 'undertake direct treatment of children under medical supervision'.[34] Of course this was in effect what was already happening in some places although the willingness to dilute the psychiatric input is striking here. But the issue of a lack of specially trained psychiatrists was real enough. Dr Alan Maberly, in 1945 Director of the Provisional National Council on Mental Health, told a conference that at present there was 'hardly anyone available to train for such a service, let alone adequate training facilities for them'. In his rather gloomy prognosis, child guidance services were thus 'bound to be inadequate for some years to come'.[35] While this was no doubt accurate enough, it is nonetheless revealing to place these remarks in the context of St Loe Strachey's complaint, noted in the previous chapter, that child guidance was being neglected by the broader mental health movement.

And as Thomson has shown, the wartime government had commissioned the psychiatrist and eugenicist C. P. Blacker to carry out a survey of existing mental health services. Blacker's plan was a 'mental hygienist design for a national mental health service', which included an expansion from mental asylums and mental deficiency institutions into the community by way of, for example, child guidance clinics and increased numbers of PSWs. This plan was, though, seen as unfeasible and the conclusion drawn that 'any large scale extension of services was in fact out of the question'.[36] Sybil Clement Brown's views on Blacker's proposals about child guidance are revealing. There was a strong argument, she suggested, 'that the first child guidance services should be available within the school system' and that this should 'cater for consultation about the ordinary needs of normal children, socially as well as educationally'. The proposed distinction between the 'child guidance centre and the child psychiatric clinic seems therefore to be a useful one, provided they are very closely related, and never allowed to become competitive'.[37] This reminds us of contemporary debates as to whether child guidance should be for the severely maladjusted or for much more frequently occurring minor problems.

This issue was to be much more problematic than Brown anticipated. Addis, in a report for the NAMH in the early 1950s, remarked on the emergence of 'two schools of thought, the protagonists of the classical child guidance clinic and those who would distinguish child guidance centres as part of the education service'. What Addis's remarks further illustrate was that, as provision became the concern of central government, so too did it require rules and definitions which had been previously unspoken while a cause of division and disagreement. Differences were, in other words, increasingly the subject of formal dispute. So, as she further shows, there was considerable debate in the mid to late 1940s about what direction child guidance should take. The Association of Education Committees, for instance, argued for a distinction between child guidance centres and clinics. The former were to ascertain which children needed treatment, which was to be provided by the latter. The idea here was that there would not necessarily, or even usually, be psychiatric input at the centres, thereby taking away the diagnostic element from psychiatrists. As Addis herself remarked, there was a 'danger here of the psychologist being encouraged to deal with problems which fall within the province of the psychiatrist'. Her position was supported by the national and professional press. As an example of the latter, Addis cited an article in the *Lancet* in 1947 which 'repudiated the child guidance centre without a psychiatrist and agreed with the NAMH in standing for the team principles [*sic*]'. Such concerns were further reinforced by a 1948 Ministry of Education circular which appeared to endorse the idea of separating out diagnosis and treatment and was later criticized by the Underwood Committee for its misleading instructions.[38]

Such proposals again provoked a strong response from supporters of the 'classical' approach. In a joint letter the NAMH and the British Paediatric Association argued that child guidance was not synonymous 'with "education" but includes the ascertainment and treatment of emotional maladjustments of children'. Educational maladjustment was the responsibility of the teacher. But 'where emotional factors are involved, proper diagnosis can only be made by a child guidance team. The psychiatrist needs the partnership of the educational psychologist as well as of the psychiatric social worker' in addition to the cooperation of teachers and paediatricians. The Ministry of Education had denied seeking to separate out diagnosis and treatment but it remained the case, Addis explained, that this was precisely what some local authorities were doing. To further compound the problem, the NHS Act had certainly given responsibility for established child guidance clinics at the Tavistock and at the Child Guidance Training Centre (the London Clinic) to the appropriate Regional Hospital Board. But it had not addressed what remained the fundamental issue – namely that it was LEAs which had the legal duty to ascertain maladjustment. Putting a brave face on matters, Addis concluded that 'Close co-operation between the medical and educational services remains the ideal'.[39]

That the location of child guidance was a contentious issue is also illustrated by events on the Mental Health Standing Advisory Committee. As Charles Webster notes, this body was one of a number set up under the NHS at the insistence of the medical profession, purportedly to fulfil a strategic role and purportedly independent. It sought, in mid-1949, an investigation into the state of the child guidance service. This was shortly after the Ministry of Education had begun setting up the Committee on Maladjusted Children, eventually appointed in autumn 1950. The Advisory Committee had, as Webster puts it, 'the idea of inviting evidence and even attendance at meetings from other departments as well as the Ministry of Health'. A memorandum entitled 'Preventive Psychiatry with Special Reference to Child Guidance', one of whose authors was Bowlby, was produced which took a clear position on the need for a unified service. Bowlby further pressed for an 'interdepartmental inquiry into child guidance, with terms of reference broader than the investigation set up by the Ministry of Education'. All this raised alarm bells in other parts of the Ministry of Health, as some assumed that Bowlby was using the issue to 'advance his case for a separate government department for children' – a revealing assumption in itself. Consequently the Minister of Health and his Permanent Secretary were directly approached with the result that the Advisory Committee was steered away from the broad-ranging investigation it sought.[40]

The problems of such territorial disputes and lack of absolute clarity about where child guidance might or should be located is illustrated by the case of Portsmouth as subsequently described by psychologist Olive Sampson. A clinic had been set up in 1938 sponsored by the local psychiatric hospital, St James's. This had been staffed by a social worker attached to the hospital and a psychiatrist with sessions taking place at the hospital and at local authority-provided premises in the city. At the end of the war the LEA appointed a full-time psychologist who helped out at the clinic but worked mostly with schools. However, although psychologists might contribute to the clinic's work, 'they were not regarded as part of their team'. Matters came to a head in 1953 when the hospital set up a Department of Child Psychiatry and it was on hospital premises that this Department's child guidance activities took place independently of the LEA. This in turn led to protests by the latter over lack of communication and duplication of effort and the beginnings of its own, purely educational, service. For Sampson this was an example of the tension between what she saw as the psychiatric approach and what she obviously saw as the real function of child guidance clinics, located in education and led by psychologists.[41]

Child Guidance and Social Reconstruction

Such problems notwithstanding, we also need to ask more broadly what proponents and practitioners of child guidance wanted out of post-war reconstruction. In the last chapter we discussed wartime visions but now we turn to post-war aspirations; aspirations articulated as social reconstruction was actually being put in place and child guidance itself was now part of the developing welfare state. Our starting point is the child guidance training manual published in 1945 and written by workers at the Manchester clinic – psychiatrist Mary Burbury, psychologist Edna Balint and psychiatric social worker Bridget Yapp. Introducing the volume, Burbury made the by now familiar arguments about the scientific basis of much child guidance work and the need for it to be in the hands of specially trained practitioners. So just as a dangerous explosion might be caused by the 'ignorant playing' in a chemistry laboratory, equally dangerous was the 'practice of playing at psychology' the difference being that 'the material ... which is liable to be destroyed or damaged is the human mind'. More specifically, with regard to children Burbury suggested that personal happiness could only be achieved and 'full service to the community rendered if an individual is an integrated personality'. Of course breakdowns occurred hence the need for services such as the clinics offered. But, she continued, Britons were

> living in times when there is talk from many quarters of reconstruction and progress. We are always fighting for freedom in some way or other, but we must first be free to accept freedom, free within ourselves without internal conflict or strife.

Parents were inclined to act either as 'dictators', which stifled initiative, or to give their children too much licence. The latter made it impossible for the child to 'choose among others, since he has never had to share'. Rather, he has 'been able always to exercise his individual rights'. For Burbury, the 'truth of happy living' lay between these extremes, for 'we are individuals in society'.[42]

Here was a return to the issue of the happy child and to the need to balance discipline and freedom and, thereby, social and individual rights. Nor would Burbury's allusion to 'dictators' have been lost on her contemporaries. As had been the case from the beginning a claim was thus being made for child guidance as a social project. But the context had changed in that this claim was now being made in the wake of the most devastating war in human history and the impending polarization of the world between communism and capitalism. Burbury's rhetoric therefore draws upon contemporary British concerns for stability, order, social integration, moderation and progress and as such she was explicitly engaging with, and contributing to, the discourse of social reconstruction. The latter also involved state intervention to establish broadly agreed social goals of which the particular case of child guidance can be seen as but one example.

Others too picked up on notions such as stability and citizenship. The CMO at the Ministry of Education remarked of child guidance that it embraced a 'far wider sphere' than that of 'the restricted field of clinics'. 'The birthright of every child', he continued, was 'the mature and stable life of a worthy citizen' which could only be realized by a 'rightful and an understanding guidance from the beginning of that life'.[43] Child guidance was thus not simply something which took place in an institutional setting. It was potentially all-pervading when children were being raised and educated – the broad social remit carried out by and for society as a whole.

MacCalman, meanwhile, was one of the speakers at the International Congress on Mental Health held in London in 1948. In a session revealingly entitled 'The Family Battle-Ground' he argued that aggression in children could be dealt with in the home against 'a background of stable affection'. In particular the early stages of development would be less inclined to produce aggression if 'a determined attempt were made to give parents some knowledge of the fundamental needs of young children', a situation which did not presently prevail. Even the worst parents encountered at child guidance clinics, MacCalman claimed, responded to 'careful influence'. There was, moreover, much evidence that 'the bad parent is better than none at all'.[44] The idea that a bad parent was better than none was part of a growing rejection in child welfare of committing children to institutions as well as the claim, with evidence derived in part from child guidance experience, that the separation of children from their parents was potentially damaging to the former's emotional and psychological development. The emphasis on stability is again notable along with that on the parental role and the desire to diminish aggressiveness in children, the last unsurprising given recent history.

The need for parents to chart a middle road between discipline and licence was further explicated in the 1950 edition of the standard psychiatric text by Henderson and Gillespie, both early supporters of child guidance. In their chapter on 'The Psychiatry of Childhood' they noted that there were parental attitudes which were especially common. These were 'the over-anxious mother and the domineering father over-keen for the progress and advancement of his son'. The latter might produce either a 'weak-kneed creature lacking in initiative' or a 'sullen, defiant and sometimes furtive individual' prone to various misdemeanours. The 'baby parent' might likewise produce 'either the same namby-pamby type, or, in turn, frank rebellion'. As evidence of the problems such immoderate behaviour might cause the authors cited the case of a young woman who had developed 'schizophrenic psychosis'. Her father had 'dandled his daughter on his knee and wrote poetry about her and with her, for her childhood and into adolescence'. To put this in context elsewhere in the same volume it was argued that child guidance clinics 'should be part of a general medical organisation'.[45]

At a broader level, but attesting to the growing influence of child guidance ideas and that of its practitioners and their input to social reconstruction, by the mid-1940s key figures were participants in official investigations into child welfare. So, for example, Sybil Clement Brown and Fildes were members of the Curtis Committee which looked into the care of children deprived for whatever reason of a 'normal home life'. In addition, Bowlby, Fox and Addis were among the witnesses. The Committee's report noted, clearly with regret, that with a couple of exceptions it had found 'very little evidence that the child guidance service had begun to play a part in helping the staff of Homes with difficult children'. The number of such clinics was at present not 'on a sufficient scale to make them readily accessible'.[46] Once more this can be seen as an official endorsement of the need for increased child guidance facilities.

Hendrick notes that the reformers of the mid-1940s looked to an 'organically conceived welfare state as an antidote to the threat of possessive individualism' wherein the emotionally healthy child would help sustain the 'emotionally healthy environment, the best single guarantor of national mental health and the place where liberal values would flourish'.[47] Discussing Bowlby's 1946 article on 'Psychology and Democracy', Mayhew sees its underlying ideological basis as the need for 'state-led application of a universalistic psychology'. This was to intervene 'primarily in familial relations, and aid in the development of children to become altruistic (but otherwise autonomous) members of society'. Such intervention could be justified 'by reference to the natural tendencies of societies to become violent, and the ability of peaceful societies to create wealth for the benefit of everyone'. All this built, Mayhew argues, on Bowlby's earlier work.[48] On this last point we have repeatedly seen throughout this volume that Bowlby did indeed draw much intellectual sustenance from his child guidance experiences. And as Porter remarks, under the 'authoritative influence' of those such as Bowlby the 'nuclear family, centred on the full-time mother' became 'the sheet anchor of psychosocial adjustment'.[49] Such analyses are endorsed by the history of British child guidance and reminders that the latter has to be seen not simply as an end in itself nor as simply concerned with children but as a project with wider social ambitions and attendant responsibilities.

The Scale of Provision in the Welfare State's First Decade

To what extent, though, did child guidance expand in terms of service provision? Staffing was, as we have seen, identified as a problem from the early days of the welfare state. The Bristol Clinic's Director, Dr R. F. Barbour, told the APSW in 1949 that, given that the school population of the city was 50,000 children, his clinic was fully occupied. His main obstacle was a shortage of staff and especially PSWs. The clinic had 'three Psychiatrists, three Psychologists but only one Psychiatric Social Worker. There should be five according to U.S. standards'.[50] The use of America as a comparator further illustrates child guidance's international dimensions. As to clinics in 1950, the NAMH listed just under 150 for England and Wales.[51] Five years later the Underwood Committee recorded some 300, most operating part-time. Of the total, around two-thirds were provided by local authorities, a 'very few' by voluntary bodies and the remainder by regional hospital boards and teaching hospitals. The last two also supplied psychiatrists to 143 local authority clinics. Nonetheless, and notwithstanding the doubling of the number of clinics over a five year period, over the country as a whole 'the existing provision is inadequate'. So, for example, of the 150 local authorities one-third had at present no child guidance service at all.[52]

Around the same time, the NAMH carried out a further survey embracing both clinics and their staffing. The former clearly varied widely in size and scope with some offering extensive services. Birmingham had two psychiatrists (including Burns), five psychologists, five PSWs, one other social worker, two remedial teachers and one remedial teacher of movement. The clinic operated at three centres throughout the city. Birmingham was therefore maintaining its leading role in child guidance established in the early 1930s. At the Tavistock's Department for Children and Parents there were three consultant psychiatrists including the Director, Bowlby. This department could also call upon an assistant psychiatrist, two psychologists, three PSWs and three psychotherapists. On the other hand, and echoing the Underwood Committee, there was overall an 'acute shortage of trained workers' which had resulted in some clinics being under-staffed.[53] The question of staffing thus exercised practitioners, public officials and voluntary bodies and despite clinic expansion and the terms of the 1944 Act, parts of the country still lacked any provision at all.

A similar picture presented itself in Scotland. It was certainly the case that the general expansion of child guidance encouraged developments, or at least in engagement, in previously indifferent parts of the country. Inverness County Council, for instance, had acknowledged the importance of child guidance in 1942. But it declined to actually put anything in place and more or less consistently refused to subscribe to voluntary bodies promoting mental hygiene and health. In 1946, though, the Council agreed to send its MOH to the conference on mental health being organized by the Provisional National Council for Mental Health and, for good measure, instructed him to visit the Department of Social Medicine in Oxford.[54] It is not clear what came of all this but the following data suggests in the short term not much. The association of mental health with social medicine is revealing, however, and returned to in the next chapter.

An SED survey from around 1952 identified twenty-seven clinics. There were also child psychiatric clinics, usually attached to general or mental hospitals, in three cities and five counties. Of the twenty-seven most were run by local authorities and what was especially notable was that twenty-five were clustered in just three places – Glasgow, Edinburgh and Dundee. Glasgow alone had twelve clinics and when combined with Ayrshire, where child guidance had developed 'as an offshoot from Glasgow', this constituted two-thirds of Scottish provision. It was also noted that in Glasgow and Ayrshire clinical work was done by teacher-psychologists and that any 'psychiatric' input came from SMOs. The teacher-psychologists also carried out home visits so that no PSWs were employed although they were in some other areas. The Glasgow and Ayrshire version of child guidance was thus a long way from the American/medical model. As to administration it was acknowledged that child guidance had both medical and educational dimensions and that this had raised a problem about which part of government should have responsibility. This problem had been 'avoided, rather than solved' by the Scottish Office's failure to clarify the position publicly, a situation exacerbated by the 'professional jealousies of psychiatrists and educational psychologists'. Privately, though, the 'central government would probably regard child guidance as essentially an educational and not primarily a health service'.[55]

This position was confirmed a few years later at a meeting between the SED and a body representing professional psychologists. An official assured the visitors that they 'were not intending to alter in any way' Scottish child guidance provision. Moreover if it was decided at some future date to have a survey on maladjusted children of the type which had recently taken place in England then 'their advice would be sought'.[56] All this both further highlights Scottish difference while raising more fundamental questions as to what actually constituted 'child guidance' and who was to carry it out.

Conclusion

Child guidance was part of, and contributed to, the emerging and developing British welfare state of the 1940s and thereafter. Pre-war trends, perceptions of the evacuation experience and advocacy by individuals and bodies inside and outside government combined to enable the inclusion of services for maladjusted children in the educational legislation of the mid-1940s. In consequence over the next decade the number of clinics and of practitioners increased. More broadly, child guidance was seen by its supporters as having a key role in post-war social reconstruction in Britain. Stability in childhood, a childhood governed by emotional moderation and moderate parenting, would in turn contribute to social stability and integration. Stable and secure families were the key to such aspirations. All this was part of an understandable desire for social harmony in the wake of the devastating upheavals of war. So far, so positive, and on one level a triumph for the small band of activists who had promoted child guidance in the 1920s and a vindication of their arguments.

But of course the situation was in reality more complex. Like other mental health services, child guidance was not prioritized in the way that, for example, the NHS was in general. As Thomson remarks, the new health service 'struggled to make psychotherapeutic services more readily available'.[57] In the particular case of child guidance this was most obviously manifested in continuing staff shortages and the still patchy nature of clinic coverage. There remained, moreover, tensions and disagreements about which profession should lead and about which children suffering maladjustment should be dealt with – those easily cured or those with deep-rooted problems. And for advocates of the medical model of child guidance there was a further concern. For the most part child guidance services were in fact in the remit not of the health services but of the LEAs. This was partly because of the example of Scotland where educational psychology had from the start dominated child guidance theory and practice. From the local authority standpoint it was also no doubt the case that employing psychologists was a cheaper option and that these professionals would be easier to control than doctors, independent contractors and highly sensitive about their status. Problems thus remained about the control, delivery and aims of child guidance. In the next chapter we therefore examine the overall situation at mid-century.

7 CHILD GUIDANCE IN BRITAIN AT MID-CENTURY: 'MORE AKIN TO MAGIC THAN TO MEDICINE'

Introduction

This chapter has five interrelated strands collectively designed to situate British child guidance some three decades after its inception. The first examines psychology's apparent victory as it sought to build on the professional and legislative advantages which had accrued in the 1940s. Second, we analyse the 1951 symposium at which child guidance psychologists and psychiatrists laid out their respective approaches. While some participants attempted to promote more collegial practice, others made little effort to conceal their scepticism about those who were clearly perceived as professional rivals. We then discuss how psychiatrists saw the way forward given their apparently beleaguered position. Many were unhappy about the course of events and continued to argue for the medical model albeit adapted to meet changing circumstances and recent disciplinary developments. But psychiatry also held certain professional advantages in that, first, some clinics continued to adhere to the medical model and, second, in that by the mid-1950s psychologists were experiencing their own crisis of confidence.

Fourth, an analysis is made of the Underwood Committee as it investigated the past, present and future of child guidance. Among the issues it tackled was the apparently widespread distribution of maladjustment. The Committee had been set up by the Ministry of Education and this, it will be argued, constrained its activities given that it essentially examined child guidance as part of the education system rather than as a broader social service. Finally, we engage with another meeting, held in 1957 in response to the Underwood Report, which in its own words sought to capture 'The Changing Scene' in child guidance. Once more, differences over child guidance's organization were highlighted as well as new trends in, especially, psychiatry. Despite its physical expansion, then, child guidance continued to be divided over philosophy, organization and practice.

The Victory of Psychology?

But to start on a positive note, while tensions between psychiatrists and psychologists were inherent in child guidance, this did not mean that collaborative work was nowhere to be found. The child psychiatrist Christopher Wardle in an historical retrospective agrees that child guidance's various advances in the post-war era 'were not accompanied by universal interdisciplinary accord and collaboration'. But he also points to LEAs seeking the assistance of the new Regional Hospital Boards for psychiatrists to work at child guidance clinics.[1] Child guidance in north Wales, meanwhile, was run by the North Wales Mental Hospital Management Committee and sought to work closely with both local health and local education bodies claiming the advantages of 'a unified comprehensive service' were efficiency, lower operating costs and the avoidance of duplicated services. The clinics involved had started operating in the late 1940s and every child referred had been examined by a psychiatrist. But it was proposed to hand over some treatment to a newly appointed psychotherapist who was also qualified as a psychologist. By such accounts here was an example of harmonious, integrated and flexible working. Nonetheless child guidance was also specifically identified as a branch of medicine.[2]

In a letter to the *BMJ* a psychiatrist attached to a clinic in rural Scotland described how the local education authority supplied the educational psychologist who saw every child, as did he. All parents were interviewed either by the psychiatrist or by the PSW and either of these might be involved in the treatment of parents. As to the child, treatment was carried out either by the psychiatrist or by the psychologist and, in a passage indicative of contemporary attitudes and the membership of the two professions, the correspondent suggested that 'the fact that one is male and the other female is an advantage when deciding the treatment roles'.[3] While not explicitly stated, the involvement of the psychiatrist in all the clinic's activities strongly suggests that it was he who was in charge.

Psychiatric social work significantly expanded in the post-war era. As the Ministry of Health recorded in 1951, since its inception in 1929 the LSE course had increased its number of students fourfold. In addition, two other universities were now offering training. This report also commented on the part played by non-governmental bodies such as the Commonwealth Fund, the CGC and the NAMH in promoting the profession. Nonetheless, and further evidence of both demand and perceived staff shortages, it was also remarked that notwithstanding post-war expansion 'only a small proportion of the vacant posts could be filled each year'.[4]

Having said all that, it was psychology which gained territory in post-war child guidance. Part of this can undoubtedly be attributed to a dearth of psychiatrists and especially those prepared to work with children. The *BMJ* reported in 1951 that an LCC committee on juvenile delinquency, which included a medical representative from the NAMH, had surveyed the capital's psychiatric services and in consequence identified the need for additional child guidance provision. This was not least because the chairman of the metropolitan juvenile courts was convinced that many children ended up before such bodies because of 'long waiting lists for child guidance clinics' – once more, supply failing to satisfy demand. It was also argued that many existing clinics were staffed by 'insufficiently trained personnel' and that even more fundamentally there was not at present 'any complete or really adequate training in child psychiatry, as the six months allocated under the existing regulations for the Diploma in Psychological Medicine are not enough'. Such staffing and training issues were hence a 'problem ... calling for urgent consideration'.[5]

The same edition carried an article by Mildred Creak, psychiatrist at the Great Ormond Street Hospital for Children and by this point a member of the Underwood Committee, which similarly noted that 'even the growing number of child guidance clinics and trained workers in child psychiatry' would be 'inadequate' to meet the situation whereby up to 1.5 per cent of all children would need 'some psychological help'. Creak thus suggested ways whereby GPs might be placed in 'the front line of attack on childhood neuroses'. She stressed that GP assistance was 'no stop-gap substitute for the fully-staffed child guidance clinic' since he would already have, for example, a good knowledge of the home environment.[6] So while stressing the medical profession's role Creak, almost certainly unwittingly, subverted the bedrock of child guidance – the clinic and its specially trained staff.

Important as the lack of psychiatrists was for the advance of psychology, other factors also came into play. One was clearly the consolidation and expansion of LEA interest in, and engagement with, child guidance services which had culminated in the legislation of the 1940s. This had identified child guidance as part of the School Medical Service and gave educational psychologists the opportunity to claim the field. All this took place in the face of misgivings and sometimes direct opposition on the part of the medical model's supporters. In addition psychology as a discipline was becoming more assertive and more professionalized. The psychologist Doris Wills recalled in a celebratory article that in 1947 the BPS had set up a subcommittee to 'consider the professional status and responsibilities of non-medical people engaged in child psychotherapy'. The Society had taken advice from Kenneth Soddy, NAMH Medical Director and, somewhat surprisingly, Bowlby. One outcome was the Provisional Association of Child Psychotherapists (Non-Medical). The creation of this body can be seen as a forerunner of the claims by a range of professions to child guidance territory. Ironically or naively Wills also remarked that 'unbelievable' as it might seem in the late 1970s, when the Provisional Association was being set up there was a motion before the LCC Mental Health Advisory Committee 'that lay psycho-therapists should not be employed in the Health Service' and that support for this was being sought from 'various august bodies'.[7]

In fact the BPS initiative described by Wills was part of a broader move-ment within psychology to establish itself in the emerging welfare state. In 1937 the Society reacted extremely defensively to a CGC request for information on psychologists' professional qualifications. By 1942, though, more positive and proactive steps were being taken. A committee was set up, with Fildes as the key figure, to look into forming an association of 'psychologists engaged in child guid-ance or educational work, and to make recommendations for the training and selection of candidates'. The BPS also initiated discussion on topics such as 'The Psychologist in the Child Guidance Clinic'. All this led to the formation in 1943 of the Committee of Professional Psychologists (Mental Health). The following year, flexing its muscles, the BPS expressed concern about a leaflet on child guid-ance training produced by the Provisional National Council for Mental Health and which appeared to imply that clinic directors should always be psychiatrists.[8]

This process of psychologists taking the opportunities afforded by social reconstruction has been analysed by Hall. For present purposes his key arguments are as follows. First, at the outbreak of the Second World War it was educational psychologists, working either with educational bodies or in child guidance clin-ics, which 'formed the most homogenous group of psychological practitioners'. Second, Hall stresses the significance of the formation of the Committee of Pro-fessional Psychologists (Mental Health) which 'implicitly assumed responsibility for all psychologists in child guidance or educational settings' or in reorganized post-war health services. The work of this body, Hall argues, was important not just in establishing training standards and salaries in negotiation with appropri-ate government ministries but also in the broader professionalization process. Its activities were hence 'foundational' for the profession. Third, although the data appear rather shaky the number of psychologists from England and Wales who were members of the Committee rose from 77 in 1945 to 350 in 1955 with most working with children or in educational settings.[9] In a relatively short period, then, psychology had gone from a position of weakness (at least outside Scot-land) to a profession with rising numbers, accepted standards of entry and a more secure place in child guidance by way of the Education Acts.

The 1951 Symposium

And with the increased assertiveness and professionalism of psychology and the growing number of psychologists engaged in child guidance came further evidence of the tensions between that discipline and psychiatry. In 1951, by which point the Underwood Committee had been constituted, MacCalman told a child guidance conference that there was a 'temperamental' distinction between the clinician and the scientist (that is, the psychologist). The latter, he suggested, was 'happier when dealing with the psychometric method, with cases as a necessary adjunct'. The 'stuff of which the great clinician' was made, on the other hand, was 'probably rather different' from that which made for a 'good scientist'. In any event the two professions had been 'remarkably rude to one another ... and I would commend to them the necessity for professional courtesy and understanding on both sides'.[10]

One important manifestation of these continuing tensions came at the symposium held at the BPS's Annual General Meeting in 1951 on 'Psychologists and Psychiatrists in the Child Guidance Service'. It was at this meeting that Catherine McCallum had outlined the history of Scottish child guidance and its longstanding dominance by psychology. Gertrude Keir, lecturer in psychology at University College London, expanded this historical approach to look at England and further afield. In both England and America there had been 'in certain quarters' a tendency to see child guidance 'as a psychiatric rather than as an educational and social task'. However, in both countries the 'narrowness of such a conception seems now to have been fairly widely realized'. So the present trend was to 'relate the problems of child guidance more closely to the general framework of psychology as a whole'. Keir was keen to trace the historic and scientific basis of modern psychology through reference to, for example, Darwin, Spencer and James Sully. Sully had founded the British Child Study Association and Keir quoted his argument that medical science was 'more familiar with the rare but striking cases of mental disease and defect'. By contrast 'mental science ... has already shown that, during childhood at least, the vast majority of cases consist of deviations within the normal range rather than aberrations from the normal' – the behavioural rather than the pathological approach already encountered in, for instance, Boyd. Child psychiatry, on the other hand, was a relatively recent development, the methods of which had been shown – by educationalists and psychologists – to be misguided and its results difficult to verify. Again this was a common and not unjustified criticism. For Keir English child guidance, unlike Scotland whose early commitment to psychology she approvingly cited, had thus initially followed the wrong path and betrayed its origins in scientific psychology. Seeking to end on a positive note, Keir remarked that while child guidance was certainly controversial and subject to a 'diversity of views', this had nonetheless resulted in 'the development of new ideas and of complementary methods of approach'.[11]

May Davidson, a psychologist from Oxford and a leading BPS member, was like Keir relatively conciliatory in tone and sought common ground while claiming that neither psychologists nor psychiatrists had all the answers. Difficulties in collaboration were likely if psychiatrists expected the psychologist to 'emulate a crystal-gazer or fortune teller' because tests and experiments 'do not provide all the answers to clinical problems'. By the same token psychologists did not regard 'tests simply as a short cut to diagnosis' but rather as 'standardised interviews which may and do prove useful in the objective study of human behaviour'. Ideally, therefore, psychologists should help psychiatrists to assess their results 'in a more objective way', while psychiatrists should assist psychologists in ensuring that the latter, in their pursuit of 'scientific knowledge', did not lose sight of the 'ultimate aim of all clinical work ... the welfare of the individual patient'.[12] Notable here, as with other psychologists' contributions, was the emphasis on psychology's scientific status, implicitly in contrast to psychiatry.

Another who recognized the complexity of dealing with maladjusted children and promoted a collaborative approach based on the acknowledgement of shortcomings in both disciplines was the psychiatrist Alexander Kennedy. He suggested that organizationally child guidance clinics should avoid 'any hierarchy which gives one member a permanent ascendancy over other fully-trained members'. Kennedy then proposed a 'dual clinic' comprised of a 'development clinic under the supervision of a psychologist' and of a 'behaviour clinic' led by a psychiatrist. This was presumably an attempt to circumvent problems of hierarchy but it also echoes earlier calls to disaggregate child guidance functions with psychiatrists focusing on acute cases. Paediatric services should be available to both clinics and social services 'partly shared'. Equally importantly there should be 'opportunities for daily contact between the staffs and for cross-referral of cases'. Dangers to such a collaborative approach included some educational psychologists' tendency to believe that 'the cause of practically all disturbances fall within their province' or to 'attempt to give psychiatric treatment because it seems to be easy enough' – a reassertion of psychiatry's specialized knowledge and primacy in diagnosis and treatment. Psychiatrists on the other hand might 'tend to interpret too large a proportion of their cases in terms of one system of thought and similarly neglect the advantages on an eclectic approach'. So while there was no need for all clinics to work in the same way, it was absolutely necessary that the form and content of professional training was set and monitored by appropriate professional bodies.[13]

Robert Moody, a London-based psychiatrist, was more robust. No preceding speaker, he commented, had 'sufficiently emphasised the tension, and at times bitterness' which had existed between psychiatrists and psychologists. Pressing the point home and employing his own psychiatric expertise, he further suggested that despite much excellent work in British child guidance's 'chequered history', behind the scenes there had been between the two disciplines 'rivalries, persecutions, over-compensations, and power-drives such as do no particular credit to anyone'. Nor was this a thing of the past. The situation was partly attributable to psychologists' 'widespread unwillingness ... to accept the limitations of their discipline'. Psychologists often paid only 'lip-service' to psychiatry, seeing it as just a 'safeguard for dealing with what have been curiously described as "definitely pathological cases" and perhaps some of the grosser forms of psychosomatic disease'. Psychiatrists were in this view clinicians whose concerns with pathology had put them 'out of touch with normal or near-normal children' and were hence unsuitable for 'dealing with the diagnosis and treatment of the everyday problems of child guidance'. It was true that child psychiatry had adopted 'much of what was first discovered and worked out by psychologists'. Equally, though, psychologists owed 'an enormous debt to psychiatry and psycho-analysis without which the psychotherapeutic treatment of disturbed children would have remained in the wilderness'. Many psychologists had, moreover, become over-reliant on 'the efficacy of superficial methods of diagnosis and treatment indiscriminately applied' and were hence uninterested in the 'deeper aspects of maladjustment'. Little wonder, then, at 'psychiatrists' insistence on medical direction of clinics where possible'.[14]

Moody too acknowledged the different situation in Scotland, remarking that there psychologists had encountered 'no competition, much less victimization, from the medical profession'. It was nonetheless revealing that Scottish child guidance was 'now becoming more conscious of the need for a consultative service of doctors trained in child psychiatry'. The position of psychologists in England had 'shown a striking contrast. For many years they were a professionally dissatisfied body, and only recently has the tide begun to turn in their favour'. However, Moody recognized that all was not well with his own profession. There were few inter-professional conflicts in situations where psychiatrists had been specifically trained in child psychiatry. The issue arose where a well-trained psychologist, used to working with children, was led by a 'psychiatric director of the clinic' lacking both the experience and knowledge of children's problems. This had resulted in much resentment by psychologists, particularly those working outside London, and the distinction between the trained and untrained child psychiatrist was fundamental to the 'mass prejudices on the part of psychologists against psychiatry'. The medical profession therefore had largely itself to blame since 'by claiming Child Guidance as a branch of medicine it incurred obligations which it had not at that time the trained personnel to carry out'. As a result of their own insecurities psychiatrists not trained in child psychiatry had been 'either ineffectual or autocratic', so compounding the problem. Moody saw the solution in better training and claimed to be relaxed about who should lead any given clinic provided all-round professional standards were achieved (he was unable to resist commenting on the 'extremely variable' quality of psychologists).[15]

If Moody was combative, so too was the final speaker, Cyril Burt. Burt started off by contrasting the factual and impartial papers of Keir, McCallum and Davidson with the 'avowedly controversial' contributions of Kennedy and Moody. Burt used purported differences between the two psychiatrists to make the more general observation that it was difficult to find 'an acceptable definition for the terms "psychiatrist" and "psychiatry"' and he highlighted as a further instance the Melanie Klein/Anna Freud dispute – not of themselves unreasonable points. Picking up on Kennedy's claim that psychiatry was a branch of medicine, Burt rolled out the now familiar argument that medicine was 'concerned primarily with illness, not with giving advice or aid to those who are neither ill nor in any danger of becoming ill'. Psychology in contrast to psychiatry was easily defined as the 'science of mental life'. Burt conceded that the term psychologist too was ambiguous and that it was necessary to distinguish between general and applied psychology, an example of the latter being those trained in educational psychology and thereby qualified to work in child guidance.[16]

Turning specifically to child guidance, Burt put forward a substantive argument which he then summarized under five key points. First, only between 10 and 15 per cent of children sent for child guidance had pathological conditions and he too quoted approvingly Sully's observation about deviations within rather than from the normal. Hence the 'essential problem' was to investigate the maladjustment, which could be of varying degrees, 'between the child's personality and the environmental conditions'. Second, analysis of case records and follow-up surveys had shown psychiatrists' diagnoses to be for the most part 'highly subjective' and in most cases less successful than those of psychologists. Third, because of their lack of proper training in psychology most psychiatrists were 'too prone to interpret normal reactions in psychopathological terms' while overlooking 'the specific psychological, educational, and social aspects of each individual case'. Psychologists' training by contrast included a 'thorough study of the whole range of individual differences' thereby making them 'far better equipped to deal with the wide variety of problems occurring in normal [i.e. non-pathological] cases'. Fourth, there was a need for both psychiatrists and psychologists in child guidance. But given that 'the majority of cases call ... for a psychologist who can train the child rather than for a physician who can diagnose and treat mental illness' then the former should be 'the key person'. Finally, outcomes currently fell 'far short of what seems possible and desirable' despite in some cases much public expenditure. There was thus an 'urgent need for more scientific research, particularly on the efficacy of different modes of treatment'.[17]

Considerable attention has been paid to the 1951 Symposium as it highlights differences between psychiatry and psychology central to understanding British child guidance's history. What, though, were the main points it illustrated? First, notwithstanding their differences of approach both psychiatrists gave a strong sense of being on the defensive. For them their profession's control over child guidance was being undermined. More than this, child guidance was being diverted from its medical foundations to an approach relying on more quantifiable, but nonetheless more superficial, techniques – those of psychology. All this clearly reflected these psychiatrists' perception of child guidance's trajectory since the 1940s.

Second, and by contrast, implicitly and explicitly the psychologists evidently felt their time had come. Child guidance in England had taken a wrong path by adopting the American/medical model but was now returning to its true psychological roots. Much was made of psychology's purportedly systematic and scientific nature in contrast to the lack of uniformity and cohesion in psychiatric thought, practice and outcomes. The medical model was, moreover, fundamentally misguided because most child maladjustment was a behavioural rather than a pathological problem.

Finally, and rhetorical bluster notwithstanding, some attempt was made to find a common ground or at least an accommodation. The otherwise combative Moody frankly and legitimately recognized his own profession's failings with respect to specialized training. It was noted too that tension between the two disciplines had its creative dimensions and that in any event different circumstances might require different approaches. There was also general agreement that professional standards all round had to be established and maintained. And the very fact that the symposium took place at all suggests a widespread acknowledgement that something had to be done about the relationship between the two professions, especially in England. Nonetheless tensions were clearly present as was, in certain individuals, an evident scepticism about the scientific or clinical claims of rival disciplines. Underlying this was the fundamental disagreement as to whether maladjustment was a behavioural or a medical problem, something difficult to resolve however well-intentioned individuals were.

Psychiatrists and Post-War Child Guidance

Psychology's position in British child guidance was without doubt considerably strengthened in the post-war era. But psychiatry was not passive in the face of this territorial expansion as Moody's pugnacious stance attests. We have encountered clinics where, collaboration notwithstanding, it was the psychiatrist who took the lead. And as the psychiatrist Aubrey Lewis rather ambiguously told the British Sociological Association in 1953:

> Extension of the doctor's province has gone very far in psychiatry ... He is nowadays often, and quite properly, asked to investigate and treat disturbances of behaviour in children which can hardly be included within any warranted conception of illness.[18]

The ambiguity and definitional problems of maladjustment and normalcy are implicit here, as is perhaps a broader concern about childrearing in complex modern societies.

In less opaque terms MacCalman told the Royal Society of Medicine in 1949 that the 'debt which psychiatrists owe to ancillary workers must be recognized' and he went on to argue that 'in the future we must devise means of using nurses, psychologists, social workers, occupational therapists and the like' to ease the psychiatrist's workload. This was not least because no new psychiatrists had as yet been appointed in the recently created NHS and indeed in the foreseeable future it might not be possible to create a 'comprehensive mental health service'. MacCalman also counselled against being seduced by 'the wave of popularity which threatens to engulf psychiatry' and 'the implied flattery of being consulted about even wider social and national problems'.[19] But the key word in these passages for present purposes is 'ancillary'. Psychologists and social workers were to be given their due and their responsibilities increased but essentially they were to remain subordinate to psychiatrists.

The chair of the Child Psychiatry Section of the Royal Medico-Psychological Association, Kenneth Cameron, told colleagues in 1955 that it was undoubtedly the case that in England psychology had laid the foundations for the development of child guidance. Nonetheless it was 'established in the field of psychiatry and medicine' and indeed Cameron claimed that its comprehensive approach – utilizing in particular medicine, social work and psychology – put child guidance in 'the unique position of being from its origins social medicine'.[20] Social medicine was very much in vogue at this time and had in common with child guidance, as Cameron suggested, a team of workers led by someone medically trained as well as an emphasis on prevention. Equally, social medicine was also concerned with what constituted the 'normal' and with the relationship between individuals and their surroundings. As John Ryle, clinician and leading figure in social medicine, put it in 1947 there was a spectrum wherein 'health and disease know no sharp boundary'. What was 'normal' in one set of circumstances might not be in others hence 'organism and environment' were indivisible. These were sentiments both widely known in medical circles and to which advocates of medically-based child guidance would have happily subscribed.[21]

The psychiatric approach to child guidance also gained support from other doctors directly involved in the field. Dr Alfred Newth, encountered in the last chapter, was Senior SMO for Nottingham. In an article entitled 'What is Child Guidance?' he summarized the history of the subject and commented on the currently unsatisfactory nature of classification. The causes of maladjustment were 'innumerable, involving social, educational, psychological, medico-psychological and medical factors interwoven very closely'. Such complexity justified the team approach. The latter was the 'essential foundation on which child guidance was built up in America, and although individual workers have had success by other methods of approach at times it can hardly be called child guidance'.[22] Given that the American model was predicated on the primacy of psychiatric medicine, Newth's position is clear and one which he had already expressed to the Underwood Committee.

And particular clinics continued to employ hierarchical teamwork underpinned by the medical model. In a retrospective account from 1959 it was noted that the Bristol clinic had tended to 'run on the older pattern of child guidance' and over time had begun to move towards a more 'medically orientated set-up' hence the 'increasing preference for the name "child psychiatry" rather than child guidance'.[23] This descriptive shift can be seen as a concern to move away from what some in the field saw as an outdated and rather restrictive approach and is dealt with further below. Manchester was another city where psychiatry continued to dominate and indeed the LEA appears to have been anxious to expand on this aspect of child guidance. So, for instance, in 1946 it was suggested that the clinic's work had 'touched the barest fringe of a very large problem' and hence that the 'provision of a Psychiatric Observance Home as an integral part of [the clinic's role] is a development which we feel should come in the very near future'.[24]

In Manchester case records, meanwhile, we find the lead role still being taken by the psychiatrist.[25] Child F, a 7-year-old girl, was seen by a psychiatrist in summer 1953. He told a member of the School Medical Service that while the home background was comfortable and the parents apparently devoted to their children nonetheless the mother gave the impression of being 'somewhat obsessional'. The child herself, who had an IQ of 123, had become reluctant to leave her mother when taken to school and during her interview the psychiatrist had learned that she had become interested in a neighbour's baby. His conclusion was thus that 'many of her present difficulties were related to her unsatisfied curiosity about family life'. She was not, though, severely disturbed and 'should do well following a few interviews, provided we can help her mother to be less anxious and formal with the child'.

Child I, an 8-year-old boy, was referred for pilfering in 1955. The mother had brought the child to the clinic where both were seen by the psychiatrist. Again it was the psychiatrist who dealt with the Education Department, telling an official that the boy was of average intelligence and the middle of three children. During the birth of his younger sister when aged four, Child I had been separated from his mother for the first time and boarded with his grandmother. The latter was 'a very domineering woman' whom the patient's mother claimed had 'made her own life difficult as a child'. Child I had a challenging relationship with his elder brother whom he felt was preferred by his parents. The psychiatrist had concluded that the pilfering was an attempt to compensate for what he perceived as his parents' disapproval and that the sweets he bought with the stolen money 'also suggests a wish to solace himself with something which reminds him of his infantile satisfaction'. A further symptom had emerged when, having been informed upon by his elder brother, Child I began bed-wetting. The psychiatrist felt that the mother, herself 'a dominating character', would accept advice but that it would be 'difficult to persuade her to adopt any radical change of attitude'. At present Child I had thus to be classified as maladjusted.

It is revealing to place these case studies, with their particular emphasis on the mother and on the need to walk a middle path between discipline and licence, in the context of broader contemporary thinking on child guidance. In the late 1940s Bowlby argued that child guidance workers worldwide had increasingly come to realize that the 'overt problem' of the child at the clinic was not the real issue. Rather, what had to be addressed was 'the tension between all the different members of the family'. Child guidance was thus concerned 'not with children but with the total family structure'. Bowlby stressed the need to engage with the father early on and illustrated this with the case of Henry, a 13-year-old boy whom he had been seeing for over two years. Henry, although intelligent, had been performing poorly at school and his general behaviour was unsatisfactory. Bowlby soon established that the problems' origins derived from his relationship with his mother. Initially, he sought to treat the boy on his own but this appeared to be going nowhere. A meeting was thus arranged where Henry was seen along with both parents. This was, Bowlby suggested, a 'very interesting and valuable session', during the early part of which all three family members aired complaints about the others' behaviour. In turn this led to a greater understanding by all three of their respective feelings. The meeting ended on a positive note with the participants agreeing to seek 'new techniques for living together' and this proved to be 'the turning point in the case'. Bowlby stressed that it was not only Henry who benefitted. In their social relations at the workplace, as well of course at home, mother and father too saw improvements. So, he concluded, 'child guidance work may be expected to contribute to more co-operative *industrial* relations' and not just those within the family. As to his own role, Bowlby likened it to that of a surgeon who 'does not mend bones – he tries to create the conditions which permit bones to mend themselves'.[26]

What is notable here is Bowlby's emphasis on the whole family, although it was the mother who was at the root of the problem. Equally, child guidance was a potentially important contributor to wider social harmony and stability and in one which the psychiatrist facilitated recovery rather than laid down prescriptive rules. As we shall see, this last point, which was pre-figured in some of the case studies in chapter 4, led to a questioning of the expression 'child guidance'. The stress on the whole family as psychiatric subject is further witnessed by the 1955 Inter-Clinic conference, entitled 'The Family Approach to Child Guidance – Therapeutic Techniques'. The papers were introduced by Bowlby who reiterated that since the end of the war 'we have spent a good deal of time studying the problem of how best to treat both children and parents, recognising that in child guidance work the treatment of the two is inextricably linked'. The family was, he suggested, a 'small group where each member inter-acts with all the others and in which powerful and primitive emotions are at work'. There was furthermore a 'narrow threshold between healthy and unhealthy interaction within a family' and hence 'relatively small shifts in the balance of forces' could have either positive or negative outcomes.[27] Once more we encounter the idea of a spectrum of health rather than a rigid boundary between health and ill-health.

Bowlby's fellow psychiatrist at the Tavistock, Dugmore Hunter, expanded on these ideas. Given familial interconnectedness it was worth asking whether the child referred to the clinic was 'really the most ill member of the family'. The child patient might have been 'forced into illness by a mother and father who for some reason must avoid awareness of disturbance in themselves and so provoke mental illness in the child'. Indeed children's mental health was highly dependent on that of their parents. Problems were exacerbated by the phenomenon of neurotic individuals tending to marry other neurotic individuals and then acting out their neuroses 'in their marriage and in their relations to their children'. Multigenerational problems were thus present in many of the cases presented at clinics. Hunter stressed the insights of psychoanalysis for child guidance practice and like Bowlby the greater attention now paid to fathers. And in common with others in the field Hunter noted that the 'traditional' approach to child guidance had been somewhat didactic and overly focused on the individual child. The very expression 'child guidance' was indicative of this approach which 'many are now discarding'. At the Tavistock the phrase was no longer used as it was misleading to 'suggest that the emphasis is all on the child or that we dispense the advice which people look for under the word "guidance"'.[28] The last point again suggests the desired move away from prescription to a psychiatric approach which encouraged patients themselves to identify the source of their problems. Bowlby agreed, albeit in a rather more moderate way, that the phrase 'child guidance' did not adequately describe what he and his colleagues did since nowadays they gave 'as much time to the treatment of the parents as to that of the children'. Indeed the underlying cause of the child's symptoms derived from a 'far more complex and often partially hidden situation in which emotional difficulties of the parents usually play a large part'.[29]

However, matters of definition and classification continued to concern child guidance psychiatrists. Returning to one of his recurrent themes MacCalman noted in 1947 that the 'growth of character and personality' was the most important 'mode of development'. But emotional development was 'subtle, capricious and ephemeral' and without 'exact methods of measurement and comparison'. Further compounding the problem was that within the child population 'individual differences are enormous'.[30] The Medical Director of the Bradford clinic, Dr Edelston, observed that in child guidance classification was 'notoriously difficult and unrewarding, and no generally accepted system, say for registration and statistical purposes, has as yet evolved'.[31] Cameron likewise pointed to the lack of clear diagnostic categories in child psychiatry. He then noted a 'distressing new element' further confusing matters – the term 'maladjusted'. In principle this was a 'neutral word' describing 'a group for whom special provision is required' but it was now being 'reified as a clinical entity'. It is hard to know exactly what Cameron meant by this comment – by 1955, when it was made, maladjustment was hardly a new term – but it may be a critical reflection on the findings of, and evidence to, the Underwood Committee which reported in the same year and to which Cameron had been a witness. However, in this article Cameron, with several qualifications, did attempt formulate a system of classification and this is summarized in Appendix 2 (p. 187–8). What is again notable here is the acknowledged lack of clarity in defining terms such as 'emotional maturity'.[32]

To sum up psychiatry's position in child guidance at mid-century, in places such as North Wales, Bristol and Manchester psychiatry had maintained its leading role. This was a notable achievement especially in the case of the last two given that child guidance was principally provided by the LEAs although it is equally important that both were well-established services with long pedigrees. The case of North Wales, on the other hand, is an example of a service built up after the war but nonetheless adopting the medical model. What seems to have been important here was the initiative taken by the local mental hospital service and its ability to work collaboratively with the education authorities. As the Manchester case studies reveal, there may have been ongoing debates and anxieties about how to define terms such as maladjustment but nonetheless psychiatrists still had no hesitation in labelling children. And while problems of definition, classification and terminology remained troublesome, the engagement with them nonetheless suggested a continuing search for answers to difficult questions. So psychiatry was, at least in certain respects, holding its own against the territorial incursions of psychology as well as seeking to advance new ideas and approaches in child guidance practice. But how did it fare in the findings of the body to which we now turn, the Underwood Committee?

The Committee on Maladjusted Children

The Committee, appointed in October 1950, reported in autumn 1955. The Report provided an opportunity for a *BMJ* leader to reflect on maladjustment. The notion of 'adjustment' was based on a 'biological standpoint that has been so distinctive a feature of British child psychology since the days of Darwin and Spencer' and took as its starting point the 'individual's relation to the circumstances and people that make up his environment'. Restating a fundamental child guidance principle, it was further asserted that the 'most influential conditions are not the material or the economic, but the personal and the social'. Clinic reports had shown that it was in the 'emotional relationships between the child and other members of his family' that the 'commonest causes of maladjustment are to be found'. Nor was this a statistically insignificant problem. While the Committee had struggled to quantify the numbers involved accurately, nonetheless its enquiries had left 'little doubt that the frequency [of maladjustment] has been greatly underestimated'. Somewhere between 5 and 12 per cent of children might be seen as requiring attention although – and the leader attempted no explanation for this – 'there were marked differences according to district and social class'. However when intervention did take place in about two-thirds of cases improvement occurred after 'suitable alterations' at home or at school.[33]

The APSW recorded that the Report 'revealed a considerable appreciation of the value of the psychiatric social worker in the child guidance clinic', that the Association had formed a discussion group to consider its implications and that it would be the subject of an impending NAMH conference.[34] In fact there were a number of conferences and meetings held on the subject by the Association or its affiliates. So the 1957 Annual Conference was devoted to the report, attended by over 900 people, opened by the Lord Chancellor and addressed by speakers including Bowlby and Creak.[35] At an earlier meeting, meanwhile, May Davidson suggested that the Report constituted a 'new landmark in the history of Child Guidance in Britain'. It was a 'clear recognition' of child guidance's role in 'helping maladjusted children' and as such had given its provision a 'firm written mandate'.[36]

So Underwood received a good press, at least publicly, from representatives of all three child guidance professions. But behind the scenes various interest groups had sought to promote their own causes. In a memorandum submitted to the Committee in 1952 the NAMH reiterated that environment caused maladjustment and hence that for the 'young child such factors as over-crowding or poverty are negligible compared with the need for satisfactory relationships'. It was also argued that each of the three professions involved should be suitably qualified and 'trained in working together as a team', for in 'well run clinics' joint case discussion and the 'sharing of treatment services' predominated. Nonetheless, only a child psychiatrist should be allowed to designate a child as 'maladjusted' and this process should be 'reserved for cases where treatment is considered necessary ie. the child has failed to respond to ordinary wise handling'.[37] Another version of this document remarked on the need for further specialist studies of maladjustment such as those by Anna Freud and Bowlby and, in its discussion of 'Child Guidance Services', affirmed that the Association held 'firmly to the principle established by the Child Guidance Council in 1929' and subsequently developed in clinics that 'for full investigation and treatment of children's problems, the three-fold approach of the child guidance team is necessary'.[38] In short, the primacy of medicine in the context of hierarchal teamwork was reasserted.

The views of SMOs were given by the professional body to which they belonged, the Society of Medical Officers of Health. Particularly striking here was Newth's evidence. In Nottingham, he explained, he felt responsible to the LEA for the proper running of the child guidance service and it was he who authorized all documents and reports with the cooperation of child guidance team members. Nonetheless Newth left all the clinic's 'technical activities' to the psychiatrist and claimed that the psychiatrists with whom he had dealt 'liked these arrangements'. On the function of the educational psychologist he chose his words carefully without hiding their ultimate meaning. It was important that each team member 'should be free to work on his own initiative'. But the psychologist should also realize that 'he was acting on behalf of the team and any action taken independently should be such as would likely be approved ultimately by the psychiatrist'.[39] Newth was clearly an individual with strong views which were not necessarily entirely in line with the rest of his colleagues. But he was a leading member of his professional organization and prepared to stand up for other branches of medicine.

The BPS agonized early on about its submission. Davidson, charged with drafting the Society's evidence, noted that there had been disagreements about the composition of the child guidance team and, in particular, about the causes of maladjustment.[40] It is not clear from the evidence what the basis of such disagreements was but what this perhaps suggests is that psychology as a profession was rather less unified than it sought to make out. Some four years later, though, there was agreement that action was needed on a proposal being discussed by the Committee. Davidson reported that the latter was going to recommend a 'considerable increase' in the number of educational psychologists through recruitment among non-graduate teachers who would be then be sent on a training course. She was charged with drafting a letter to the Committee explaining that 'while the need for additional Assistants in the Child Guidance Service was recognised' anyone recruited in the proposed manner would not meet the BPS's requirements for associate membership and thus 'should not be known as psychologists'. Instead, training facilities for 'fully qualified' educational psychologists should be expanded.[41]

The Royal Medico-Psychological Association subsequently noted that its evidence to the Committee in 1952 had expressed regret that the issue was seen as solely in the remit of the education system and by 1958 its view was 'more emphatic'. The Committee's terms of reference, it concluded, had 'seriously limited the usefulness of the ... Report as contributing to the planning of services to help the emotionally disturbed child'.[42] Against this background of competing professional claims what was the Committee's remit, who were its members, who gave evidence and what were its principal findings?

The Committee was set up with a brief to 'enquire into and report upon the medical, educational and social problems relating to maladjusted children, with reference to their treatment within the educational system'. It reported five years later to the Minister of Education, David Eccles. Eccles noted that this was a unanimous report which had 'covered much ground and ... made many interesting suggestions' although he was non-committal about how many would actually be implemented. The Committee had seventeen members and was chaired by Dr J. E. A. Underwood, in 1950 Principal Medical Officer at the Ministry of Education. Among its other members were Sybil Clement Brown, now at the Home Office, and the two wartime visitors to Scotland who had been persuaded of the need for a psychological approach to child guidance, Dr Alford and Mr Lumsden. As a whole the Committee was dominated by educationalists or individuals attached to the Ministry, although nearly half were also medically qualified. The Committee members most inclined to support the 'medical model' were probably Brown, Creak, Dr H. M. Cohen (Birmingham's Principal SMO) and possibly Dr Alfred Torrie. Torrie was Medical Director of the NAMH although he appears to have had little to do with child guidance.[43] To put it another way, the fact of being organized by the Ministry of Education and its remit and composition almost certainly predisposed the Committee towards a psychological rather than a psychiatric approach to child guidance, the point forcibly made by the Royal Medico-Psychological Association.

The Committee took evidence from over thirty organizations, eight LEAs and twenty-seven individuals. Included in the first category were the BMA (representatives included MacCalman), the BPS (representatives included Burt and Davidson), the NAMH (representatives included Bowlby and Addis) and the Royal Medico-Psychological Association (representatives included Cameron and, again, Bowlby). Educational bodies such as the Association of Education Committees also gave evidence, as did the Magistrates' Association. Among the points made by the latter were that child guidance clinics were of value to the courts but that there was not enough of them, that there should be an 'earlier recognition' of maladjustment and that there should be 'more positive education for parenthood and psychiatric help should be given to mothers attending infant welfare clinics'.[44] The evidence of the LEAs was focused on the level of maladjustment and among these were Birmingham, Somerset (whose representatives included Frank Bodman) and Berkshire; their surveys are discussed below. Individuals giving evidence included the course leaders for psychiatric social work at the LSE and at the University of Manchester.[45]

The Report itself made just under a hundred recommendations, of which around half dealt with various forms of residential care and are thus not considered here. One of the key proposals, as might be anticipated, was that the clinic-based child guidance service should be significantly expanded over the coming decade. The optimum ratio of the respective professions was that for every psychiatrist there should be two educational psychologists and three PSWs. This would involve a numerical expansion from 56 to 140 psychiatrists, 141 to 280 educational psychologists and, most strikingly, 109 to 420 PSWs. And as noted the Committee also commented on the absence of any child guidance service in around one-third of local authorities. Such a level of expansion was deemed a 'comparatively modest objective' and it was stressed that this 'ten-year objective is in no sense an attempt to forecast ultimate requirements'.[46]

This last point in turn reflected a central problem for the Committee – esti-mating the 'size of the problem'. It is notable that implicit in this is the belief that a problem existed in the first place. But it was acknowledged that maladjust-ment was a slippery concept and that there were challenging methodological and definitional issues involved. Early on in the Report, for example, it was sug-gested that normal development in childhood was ideally 'development towards independence, stability and control, and the gradual drawing together and realization of all a man's [sic] capacities' – once more, the desire for emotional moderation and restraint. But it had to be recognized that the word 'normal' was problematic and that a 'criterion of normality is peculiarly difficult to obtain'. This was because, for instance, every child was unique and what was 'normal' in one might not be so in another. Similarly, 'normal' behaviour should not neces-sarily be equated with 'good' behaviour – again, circumstances were important. The 'destructiveness' of a maladjusted 10-year-old was very different from the 'dispassionate destructiveness' of a normal 2-year-old. In the latter's case he was simply engaging with the material world in an attempt to understand it better.[47] Here we have further evidence of the influence of the psychology of individual difference alongside the need to locate the child in its particular circumstances.

Early attempts at estimating the level of maladjustment among the entire child population had been abandoned and instead surveys had been carried out in Somerset, Berkshire and Birmingham. The Somerset survey sampled just under 900 schoolchildren. Head teachers filled out questionnaires, the data from which was analysed by the three educational psychologists running the enquiry. The latter then interviewed children deemed to be maladjusted by school staff or psychologists and visited the homes of around 80 per cent of the children concerned. On the basis of these investigations it was calculated that nearly 12 per cent of children sampled were 'very maladjusted' or 'probably mal-adjusted', with the former 'needing special treatment by a child guidance clinic team'. The same categories were used in the Birmingham and Berkshire surveys and these suggested equivalent proportions of 7.7 and 5.4 per cent respectively. The Report also cited other estimates. The Scottish Advisory Council on Educa-tion had worked out in 1952 that in planning for the education and treatment of maladjusted children it should be assumed that they constituted some 5 per cent of the school population. Alarmingly, a survey carried out by a psychiatrist at the Tavistock in the late 1940s of 8-year-old male pupils in a London primary school had found an incidence of maladjustment of between 35 and 42 per cent while a survey of young males presenting themselves for National Service, again in the late 1940s, had purportedly uncovered a very similar proportion.[48] Even if the more modest levels suggested by the local authority surveys were more accurate there clearly existed a significant problem for those concerned with the nation's mental health, both in the present and in the future.

An expanded service should also be encouraged to work with other child welfare agencies such as maternal and infant welfare clinics since it was now 'increasingly held that the most serious emotional damage is often done before the child reaches the age of five or even before the age of two' – this almost certainly reflects the evidence and impact of Bowlby by this point. So many of the problems encountered by the education authorities were present when the child first attended school and closer coordination of services was thus needed to address maladjustment as early as possible.[49]

More immediately, parents were in the front line of prevention for they were in the 'best position to see the first signs of emotional disturbance'. And, of course, there was 'much evidence that failure in personal relationships is the most important factor in maladjustment'. But parents faced a difficult challenge. There had never been a historical era when 'more was known about children' but in which 'parents had less confidence in their own powers to handle their children'. Parents had previously relied on 'instinct and common sense' but 'in the complexity of modern civilisation these are overlaid or mistrusted'. Popular psychology books were 'no substitute'. And of course spotting maladjustment was not always easy. Using a familiar example, the Report affirmed that maladjusted children were not necessarily unruly – on the contrary, 'some of those who are most severely maladjusted are quiet and passive'. And there was a further concern in that many people were 'ignorant and apprehensive' about what went on in a child guidance clinic seeing 'its procedures as more akin to magic than to medicine'.[50]

Underpinning the attack on maladjustment was the need for a more 'positive approach to mental health' and a shift in emphasis from cure to prevention. Such an approach was essential since 'the surest way to prevent maladjustment from arising in children is to encourage in every possible way their healthy development, particularly on the emotional side'. Addressing the difficulties for parents it was suggested that social services such as child guidance were there to help parents 'to understand and handle their own children' while not undermining parental responsibility. All children up to the age of 18, whether in education or not, should have the right to child guidance diagnosis and treatment and their parents should be allowed full access to clinics. Furthermore 'the fundamental importance of the family as a whole' should always be borne in mind so that 'action designed to keep the family together should be regarded as one of the most important aspects of prevention'.[51] This echoed MacCalman's argument that a bad parent was better than no parent.

What of the vexatious issues of organization and leadership? The Committee was careful to point out that with respect to child guidance clinics its terms of reference dealt only with actual or potential LEA provision although it did feel that its findings would 'apply in any area where the clinics in the child guidance service were provided by the regional hospital board'. The Report also urged cooperative working between education and health services. Psychiatrists' salaries should ideally be met by Regional Hospital Boards while those of educational psychologists and PSWs came from local education authorities – the issue of cost again. Predictably much was made of teamwork and cooperation, the distinct roles played by the three professions and the need for proper professional training.

But nowhere was the question of leadership addressed. Indeed it seems to have been deliberately avoided. The closest hint of inter-professional rivalries came when it was remarked that there had been debates around whether it was acceptable for 'somebody who is not medically qualified to select children for reference to a clinic'. But if child guidance was to be the 'broadly-based and comprehensive service such as we recommend' then 'this question should not need to be asked or answered'. Everyone who came into contact with children and not least parents 'carries out some child guidance in the wider sense and some selection'. And notably moving from the general to the particular the Report continued that 'if the dual role of the educational psychologist in schools and clinics is accepted' then there could be no objection 'to his taking the responsibility for deciding for many of the children whose troubles come to light in and through schools whether they need to be investigated by the whole clinic team'.[52]

Five points stand out in the Committee's findings and argument. First, it is taken as given that there was a problem of maladjustment and that this was primarily due to a dysfunctional relationship with their parents rather than, say, socio-economic circumstances. Underpinning this was the by now familiar concern with the stresses of modernity which had impacted on parents and children alike. Instinct and common sense had, the Committee rather disingenuously suggested, also been among modernity's victims. The centrality of the family was emphasized as both the best place to raise children and as a social institution. Parents should therefore have available to them the services of child guidance professionals to help them successfully negotiate their children's emotional and psychological development. Second, maladjustment was a problem on a significant scale for children, their families and society as a whole and one which necessitated a positive, preventive and sometimes interventionist approach to the nation's mental health.

Third, this consequently required much enlarged child guidance provision employing properly trained staff. While all three professions should be increased in number, the proposed expansion in PSWs was especially notable, a further example of their perceived centrality to the team and to child guidance generally. In arguing this case the Committee also drew attention to the uneven distribution of child guidance services. Fourth, the Committee avoided the leadership and organization issue, notwithstanding the debates and disagreements of which it cannot have been unaware and indeed was raised in some of the evidence submitted. Finally, and leading on from the previous point, the Committee was constrained by its remit – especially that it examine the treatment of maladjusted children within the educational system – and the fact that it was sponsored by the Ministry of Education. Of course the Committee was hardly to blame for this, nor on one level was the Ministry. Both simply did what was required of them within their respective boundaries. Nor should we ignore the behaviour of the Ministry of Health which had pushed the Mental Health Advisory Committee away from the detailed examination of the child guidance services desired by Bowlby. Overall, though, an opportunity was lost for a broad-ranging enquiry into maladjustment and child guidance. Such an enquiry might have resolved, or at least addressed more openly, inter-professional rivalries and whether child guidance was ultimately an educational or a medical service. As it was these rivalries and confusions remained.

'The Changing Scene'

Nonetheless the Underwood Report could not unreasonably be construed as a further vindication of a child guidance service driven by psychology rather than psychiatry. Once again, though, matters were not as straightforward as they might appear. At a1957 child guidance conference – called in response to the Underwood Report and revealingly entitled 'The Changing Scene' – representatives of each of the three professions contributed. Introducing the published conference proceedings Kay McDougall, senior tutor on the LSE Mental Health course and NAMH official, gave an initial sense of what this change involved. New professions were entering the field, it had become apparent that workers' roles varied from clinic to clinic and 'a number of clinics had moved a long way from the classical team of three, the psychiatrist, psychologist and psychiatric social worker all making their rather clearly defined contribution to diagnosis and treatment'.[53]

In her paper Dr E. M. Bartlett, an educational psychologist, remarked that in child guidance hers was 'the least well defined' profession, that partly as a result there were on occasions 'tensions between the members of the team' and that in turn 'psychologists are sometimes not very popular'. This was in some measure attributable to lack of clarity in psychologists' training especially when compared with PSWs. Dr Bartlett did have some positive points to make about psychologists in child guidance and their claims to specialist knowledge. So, for instance, to her it was obvious that a psychologist should 'not limit her interests to the intellectual functions of the child', another assertion of the longstanding claim that that the profession did, and should do, more than administer psychometric tests. Indeed their function had become more demanding and challenging as child guidance had developed and this was all to the good. Her overall tone was nonetheless defensive and tentative. Dr Bartlett sometimes wondered 'whether it isn't just professional arrogance on our part to say that we can prevent maladjustment'. Such was the 'incidence of emotional and neurotic difficulties' that not all children could receive the full child guidance treatment, further evidence of the perceived scale of the problem. Her concluding remark was that psychologists wished to remain in the 'full-clinic set up, we want to have the help and the guidance of the psychiatrist and the psychiatric social worker'. If this ceased to be the case then 'I think we shall not be able to continue to do our work'.[54]

This last remark in the first instance alludes to the tensions which Bartlett herself had identified and which were implicitly about child guidance's organization and leadership. But her speech as a whole is indicative of a broader trend identified by Wooldridge, who remarks that the expansion of psychology coincided with 'the spread of introspection and self-criticism within the profession'. Specifically on child guidance and individual therapy, he continues, its efficacy and approach came to be widely questioned. As the educational psychologist Jack Tizard, later Professor of Child Development at the Institute of Education, put it in 1955 and probably voicing the opinion of many of his colleagues, the whole child guidance project was essentially 'wrongly conceived'.[55] It was ironic that just as child guidance was offering an opportunity for psychologists they themselves began to question its value and their own role in it.

Back at the 1957 conference the psychiatrist Dr G. Stewart Prince made a plea for the utilization of more psychotherapy in child guidance both for individual children and for family groups. Of course psychotherapy was a field claimed by others than just the medically trained, but Prince's argument was fundamentally based in medicine. He called for a more analytic strategy and noted that what he described as the 'orthodox psychiatric approach', modelled on somatic medicine, had focused on 'fact-finding, history-taking and mental and physical examination'. All this was designed to produce a diagnosis and derived from the 'Meyerian Psycho-biology' which had had such a profound influence on British child psychiatry. But this approach was now becoming outdated. The alternative, he suggested, was 'begotten by psychoanalysis out of casework' and designed to 'meet the needs of the patient rather than those of the examiner'. Prince claimed that such procedures would enhance both therapy and 'diagnosis in depth'.[56] Psychiatry too, then, was changing and questioning its previous assumptions. For some, such as Prince and Hunter, child guidance needed to move to analytically based diagnosis and treatment. For others, such as Cameron, greater emphasis should be placed on the social medicine approach. And here we might note Wardle's later judgement that while the techniques initially employed by child guidance had been 'excellent', by the mid-1950s they had nonetheless 'become stereotyped'.[57] In whatever direction psychiatry was moving, though, it was unlikely to prove congenial to the introspective and critical mood among psychologists.

In fact Prince picked up on this last point. Bartlett, he claimed, had been 'too humble'. In a rather patronizing passage he suggested that there was no reason why a psychologist should not make diagnoses provided 'she is working in an atmosphere where skills are shared and experience is pooled'. Prince made a great deal of collaborative endeavour, arguing that flexibility was 'highly desirable but only possible where the inter-staff relationships are sufficiently secure to permit a departure from traditional roles'. But there can be little doubt that he saw child guidance as basically founded on psychiatric medicine. He concluded that the claim that we are 'passing through an epoch of change' was justified and cited Cameron – his former teacher – approvingly to the effect that there were no grounds for complacency in the present state of child psychiatry.[58] Once again the use of the expression 'child psychiatry' rather than 'child guidance' in this last passage may be indicative of the reformulated approach so forcibly expressed by Hunter.

The broader context is significant here. In the 1950s, an era of a rising number of psychiatric patients, the question of how to deal with mental ill-health was again under discussion. The most obvious manifestation of such debates was the Royal Commission on Mental Illness and Mental Deficiency (1954–7) one outcome of which was the 1959 Mental Health Act. And while Hugh Freeman correctly notes the contemporary vogue for 'social psychiatry' – he sees child guidance as covered by this definition and one of its earliest manifestations, a position similar to Cameron's – it was also an era when new drug therapies were emerging. One consequence of the latter, Long comments, was that clinical and organic psychiatry was gaining in strength. It could be argued that such diversity was a sign of intellectual rigour and engagement and it is revealing that both Freeman and Long see the coming of the NHS as an opportunity for British psychiatry.[59] But the wide variety of post-war approaches to psychiatric medicine might also be seen as sending out confusing messages especially with respect to such an inherently unfocused field such as child guidance. This can have done little to reassure sceptics and was used by critics such as Burt to attack the medical model supported by psychiatrists such as MacCalman and Bowlby.

But what of the profession that the Underwood Report had seen as in need of the greatest numerical expansion, psychiatric social work? PSWs were the single largest group to attend the 1957 conference, a reflection of both existing staff ratios and of their professional ambitions. The profession's representative, M. R. Barnes, made three notable points about what she perceived as changes in child guidance approach and provision. First, and very much in line with the Underwood recommendations, she suggested that perhaps the greatest change from the pre-war situation was 'the recognition that the ultimate success of the Child Guidance Service lay in the education of public attitudes towards mental health'.

Here she described her own post-war experience in an (unnamed) town where she had encountered considerable hostility, with one local GP suggesting that in twenty years of practice he had 'never come across a maladjusted child'. It was only through educational work and the actual benefits derived from the existence of a clinic that after five years attitudes changed from negative to positive.[60] Here we see again evidence of the continuing struggle to get the child guidance message across, even to medical practitioners.

The first of the other major changes Barnes noted was that among senior PSWs a number had gone on to take further training in psychotherapy and as such were a 'great loss to the profession'. Second, among those who remained many saw a 'greater flexibility of role between the members of the team than previously'. The psychiatrists alongside whom they worked were

> much less inclined to see them as fact-finders and more prepared to accept that information in the social history may have to be foregone in the interest of the PSW's need to build up a good relationship with the parent.[61]

This point about professional clinical interdependence had been argued by Prince and was picked up by others. Addis remarked that the PSW's role was 'complementary to, yet distinct from, that of the psychiatrist'. Put simply, the latter dealt with 'factors which work from within outward' in the patient while the PSW approach was from the 'outer factors', although of course both professions were fundamentally concerned with the effects of all factors on particular individuals.[62]

Conclusion

The title 'Changing Scene' for the 1957 conference thus seems accurate with, for instance, new occupations engaging with child guidance and with psychotherapy appearing to offer an entry for groups drawn from diverse (and not necessarily compatible) professional backgrounds. The three principal professions, moreover, were engaged in self-assessment and a reappraisal of their roles. Psychology appeared to have won the day as the rising and lead profession in child guidance, a position implicit in the Underwood Report, only to engage in a form of introspection which even asked whether much could be done for the maladjusted child and whether, indeed, child guidance was a project worth pursuing at all. Psychiatry on the other hand was both exploring new intellectual avenues and beginning to question whether its early child guidance techniques – and even the expression 'child guidance' itself – were any longer applicable. Hunter's advocacy of psychoanalysis – specifically rejected by earlier child guidance psychiatrists – and Bowlby's view of the psychiatrist as a facilitator rather than someone who handed down a rigid treatment regime are especially notable here. Psychiatry had nonetheless lost ground to psychology in child guidance organization and practice and tensions and disagreement remained between the two disciplines. PSWs, meanwhile, had seen their work endorsed by the Underwood Report and exhibited a new sense of self-confidence about their place in the child guidance team. The latter was from their standpoint enhanced by the changed attitude on the part of the psychiatrists with whom they worked.

More broadly child guidance remained a troubled project. There was still a lack of clarity about what it sought to achieve, how it was to be organized and around which profession and what its actual outcomes might be. Such problems had, of course, been present from the beginning. But, with the embedding of child guidance in the post-war welfare state, the need for clarity had become even more pressing and this was something which it was ultimately unable to offer or achieve. In the next and concluding chapter we therefore examine the major themes in the history of British child guidance from its origins in the 1920s down to the mid-1950s and draw up a balance sheet of its successes and failures.

CONCLUSION: 'THE DANGEROUS AGE OF CHILDHOOD'

Introduction

In the late 1950s the Royal Medico-Psychological Association observed that in child guidance's early days the roles of the psychiatrist and the educational psychologist were clearly distinct and seldom overlapped. As both professions became increasingly concerned with the 'whole child', though, so boundaries became blurred. But few educational psychologists had been trained 'to allow them to be competent in the therapeutic field, or to interview parents about emotional disturbances in their children'. The present shortage of child psychiatrists, however, had encouraged psychologists 'to take on quite seriously disturbed children'. This, the Association felt, 'should not be allowed to prejudice the development of a proper child psychiatric service'. Nonetheless it was certainly the case that no 'one agency can deal with a child in all its aspects'. The field therefore had to be broken up into 'functional units, of which child psychiatry is one'. Recalling a trend we noted in the last chapter it was then suggested that the term 'child guidance' was now becoming 'outmoded' and that it was thus 'more appropriate to speak of the investigation, diagnosis and treatment of disturbances in children' as 'child psychiatry'.[1] For the Association, then, child guidance as originally conceived had outgrown itself while some of those purporting to practice it, educational psychologists, were not equipped to do so.

Seven years later the NAMH remarked that child guidance was an 'anomaly in traditional medical clinical practice', that there remained a lack of systematic training in child psychiatry and that services 'for disturbed children are at a critical phase because of their inability to meet the increasing demands made by the community'. Given the potential range of sources of such disturbances all aspects of the child's life – personal, familial, social and educational – had to be taken into account and it was not within the 'competence of any one discipline to be expert in all aspects of the child's life'. The child psychiatrist therefore and 'in common with many other medical specialists' had to accept 'the professional competence of his non-medical colleagues in their own fields'.[2] Ten years after the Underwood Report, it appeared, child maladjustment still posed a problem – indeed an increasing problem – for the nation's mental well-being, child psychiatrists were still not being adequately trained and there remained the question of inter-professional boundaries. It is nonetheless also revealing that, by this account, child guidance remained primarily a branch of medicine.

Taken together these sources highlight problems which, it has been argued in this volume, were inherent in child guidance from its earliest years. But they suggest too the complexity of child guidance's aspirations and thereby bring into question the degree to which it succeeded. Of course in terms of actual provision, and while its proponents always wanted more, the first three decades or so of child guidance's existence had seen a remarkable expansion from a handful of clinics in the 1920s to its incorporation in the post-war welfare state. And, although far from uncritically received, the child guidance message had been widely broadcast and had gained acceptance among certain sections of the medical, social work and educational professions, by government ministries and agencies and by the general public by way of, for instance, Bowlby's influential work and popular journals such as *Mother and Child*. Nonetheless, child guidance was clearly also problematic, not least for its practitioners. This concluding chapter identifies six major themes in its history down to the mid-1950s and attempts to draw up a balance sheet of its strengths and weaknesses.

The American Model

Our first theme concerns British child guidance's origins and early development. Although certain qualifications are made later in this chapter, American ideas, practices and funding were clearly of huge significance. American influence had a number of aspects. First, there was the creation of child guidance clinics in the US in the immediate aftermath of the First World War. In general these were structured in such a way that the medically trained psychiatrist was the lead figure with psychologists and psychiatric social workers thereby in subordinate roles. This was the American, or medical, model of child guidance which had been financially supported and promoted by the Commonwealth Fund. Second, at the request of its British supporters the Fund extended such support by way of its English Mental Hygiene Program. This allowed for the setting up of the LSE Diploma in Mental Health – crucial to the development of psychiatric social work in Britain – as well as financing the Child Guidance Council and its various activities. Third, the Commonwealth Fund also committed resources to support the various observational and training visits to the US and probably the most crucial were those by potential or actual PSWs, child guidance's front-line workers.

Of course, and as with most cases of the movement of social reform ideas and practices across national boundaries, child guidance did not come out of the blue or into a context without local precedents. Some moves had been made towards instituting clinics by the late 1920s. Those in East London and at the Tavistock are the most obvious examples. But we have also encountered institutions which were retrospectively to claim to have been among the forerunners of British child guidance, were also established in the 1920s and explicitly rejected any American influence – the psychological clinics in Glasgow and Edinburgh. All of these were important as were the contributions of, especially, Burt to a greater understanding of issues such as delinquency, individual difference and maladjustment. British child guidance was to follow its own path too in its interwar rejection of psychoanalysis and its adoption of play therapy.

But it is hard to get away from the Commonwealth Fund's impact and in particular its promotion of the medical model. This was acknowledged by those who broadly adhered to such an approach, by those who went along with it for financial reasons rather than through any strong commitment and by those opposed to a predominantly psychiatric orientation to child maladjustment. In the first category are psychiatrists such as Moodie and MacCalman as well as official committees such as that on social work in the mental health services in the early 1950s. Into the second category fall individuals such as Sister Marie Hilda, herself trained in psychology but nonetheless prepared to conform to the medical model in order to gain Fund financing. The third category would embrace psychologists such as Boyd. Boyd was convinced not only that child guidance had, at least in England, taken the wrong direction but been paid considerable amounts of money to do so, resources denied those unwilling to conform to the American model. Such resentment was to have a long shelf-life within certain branches of psychology.[3]

Environment and Maladjustment

Our second theme involves maladjustment and its causes. A fundamental premise of psychiatrically oriented child guidance was that maladjustment derived from a malfunctioning of familial relationships and that this led to underlying pathologies which in turn outwardly manifested themselves in symptoms presented by the child. Such an analysis thereby rejected factors such as the family's socio-economic circumstances. The broader context was not entirely ignored but was seen in terms of, for instance, the psychic strains induced by modernity rather than more prosaic, material factors. This focus on the family derived, it was stressed, from science rather than morality and sought to understand the whole child in the situation by which it was most influenced. Children, and later their parents, were emotionally or psychologically disturbed rather than malicious or bad. Of course, and once again, qualifications are necessary in that, for instance, many PSWs were all too aware of local socio-economic conditions and could draw on their previous experience as more traditional social caseworkers in addressing particular problems. Similarly, some psychiatrists came to see child guidance as a sub-branch of social medicine which by definition engaged with individuals in their wider social circumstances and not simply that of the family. Nonetheless the emphasis on the family's emotional landscape persisted in much of child guidance throughout the period under discussion and so influenced the nature of both diagnosis and treatment.

Again from the standpoint of psychiatrically oriented child guidance, maladjustment was an ever-present threat even to the most apparently normal child, normalcy and abnormalcy themselves being located on a spectrum rather than being clinical absolutes. Constant vigilance was required by parents, teachers and society as a whole to prevent children from becoming maladjusted, a condition which, if not addressed, would lead to unhappiness now and in the future and contribute thereby to social instability. Childhood therefore became pathologized – as noted in the introductory chapter, such an analysis led the psychiatrist Ronald Gordon to identify 'The Dangerous Age of Childhood'. Those who proposed child guidance services based on psychology rather than psychiatry argued, by contrast, that very few children had serious psychological or emotional problems. Maladjustment was a behavioural rather than a medical problem and was generally a healthy response to environmental imbalance. Adjustment could hence be brought about relatively easily through correcting the problem in the environment. But, once more, environment was the key and maladjustment a threatening reality.

Defining the Problem, Measuring the Outcomes and Employing Resources

All this assumed a cluster of conditions which constituted maladjustment and this brings us to our third theme – definitions, classifications and resources. Clearly there are behaviours which parents, adult society in general and children themselves find challenging or disturbing. In what follows it is not being denied that these can have an impact on the lives of individuals and their families and may require some form of intervention. Nonetheless there is a strong case that at least some of what are at any given chronological point construed as unacceptable behaviours are socially and historically constructed. Discussing a widespread concern of the late twentieth and early twenty-first centuries, ADHD, Rosenberg suggests that however many 'well-conceived epidemiological studies' are carried out this will not create a 'consensus with regard to children exhibiting a problematic restlessness; it is at some level a problem of human diversity, of social class, of gender, and of bureaucratic practice'.[4] Analysis of this sort can be extended to some of the conditions we focused on earlier in this volume such as shyness and timidity, opaque clinical categories at best. And to these we could add, for instance, the 'appropriate' level of sexual activity in which a child might engage.

The lack of clarity about definitions and classifications notwithstanding, child guidance was not only willing and prepared to intervene in family situations. It was also highly labour intensive and absorbed resources from, in its early days, American as well as indigenous philanthropy and later from the state, although as we shall see below this last point is in fact rather problematic. Of course this could be justified on the basis that child mental health was indeed precarious and that the number of maladjusted children, as suggested by the surveys carried out for instance for the Underwood Committee, constituted a significant proportion of the total child population. But in fact many child guidance professionals openly and honestly acknowledged that they might indeed devote a considerable amount of time and effort to an individual child while the measurement of, most notably, emotional states was beyond the state of scientific understanding as it then existed. None of this, though, constrained practitioners from labelling children as maladjusted on what often appears to have been flimsy clinical bases. In addition we have the sort of normative judgements about behaviour encountered in earlier chapters, particularly although not exclusively in the reports of PSWs. And, as with many related aspects of welfare policy, there has historically been an elision whereby families with problems are turned into problem families. It is revealing, then, that the very concept of the 'problem family' emerged in the 1940s partly spurred on, like child guidance, by the impact of evacuation.[5] There were, in short, definitional problems as to what constituted maladjustment and thereby who was suffering from it.

More than this, though, there are questions around the outcomes of the clinical encounter where once again there were definitional and classificatory problems. If it was unclear what constituted maladjustment then this suggests that data claiming improvement or adjustment have to be viewed with a degree of suspicion. However even if it is accepted that improvements occurred, a legitimate question was posed by those suspicious of psychiatrically oriented child guidance – and even some partly supportive of it – namely would such improvements have happened anyway with either less intervention or even with none at all? Clearly this would not have been the case with those with severe psychoses but they were not by and large dealt with by child guidance clinics in the first place. Why children became patients, how they stopped being patients and quantifying how much effort had been usefully employed was thus not as straightforward a matter as it would superficially appear.

Professional Practices

Our fourth theme leads on from the last and raises the issue of what child guidance professionals actually did and how they interacted. At least in its medical version British child guidance, borrowing from its American counterpart, operated on the basis of hierarchical teamwork. Much was made of the claim that it sought to deal with the individual patient as a total entity and hence that social, psychological and medical inputs were required. As we have already noted, the 'social' in fact embraced only the child as it related to others and particularly to its parents – socio-economic circumstances were not deemed relevant. Nonetheless there was a clinic-based team which utilized case conferences to exchange specialized professional knowledge and to come to a purportedly rounded diagnosis of the patient's ailment and hence necessary treatment.

But in principle at least it was a team led by the psychiatrist. This was, from early on, resented by psychologists who had their own aspirations to clinical practice. There is also evidence that PSWs bridled at what they viewed as the psychiatrist's over-dominant role, seeing their own contribution as not simply as assistants to psychiatrists but as having active treatment responsibilities as well. In reality, this was precisely what happened given that, for the most part, psychiatrists would only see children for relatively brief periods and always in the clinic setting although it should be stressed that they continued to see themselves as at the apex of the hierarchical team. Psychologists too confined their activities to the clinic, at least outside Scotland. It was thus the psychiatric social worker who spent most time with the child and its family, both at the clinic and at home.

Over time the initially rather rigid boundaries began to shift with, for instance, both psychologists and PSWs taking on tasks relating to play therapy and various other dimensions of diagnosis and treatment. The ongoing shortage of psychiatrists able and willing to undertake child guidance work contributed to such slippages as did the emergence, after the Second World War, of other occupational groups with a claim to the field. Add to this the openly acknowledged differences in practice between clinics and the widespread rejection of the medical model in Scotland and we have further reasons why a lack of clarity existed about what child guidance was, what it sought to do and who should be doing it.

As to the actual content of each profession's contribution, psychiatric social workers saw themselves – and again the American example was important here – as among the elite of the social work profession. In terms of formal training this was at the time the case and there can be little doubt that social work was professionalized in part because of the emergence of the PSW. Nonetheless the question 'what was psychiatric about psychiatric social work' is a not unreasonable one. PSWs did, of course, engage in forms of treatment. In particular they alerted parents to perceived misjudgements and faults in the way they were bringing up their children and this may have been informed by the social work-er's exposure to various medico-psychological theories during training. But this is difficult to show and most PSWs' case notes employ little in the way of psychi-atric language. Instead they are largely descriptive of family circumstances and as such were used at case conferences where any meaningful psychiatric input would have come from the psychiatrist. And, the relative sophistication of their training notwithstanding, the time devoted to theoretical approaches was rela-tively limited. In short, PSWs were almost certainly for the most part engaged in an updated and more sophisticated version of what nonetheless essentially remained social casework.[6]

Psychologists saw themselves as having a much greater role in child guid-ance than the medical model allowed but theirs was a rather curious history. Outside of Scotland they were, in principle at least, at first confined largely to psychometric testing, although of course this was of itself important in helping to establish the 'normalcy' of clinic patients, as was the development of ideas around individual difference. As psychology professionalized, especially from the late 1930s, this encouraged psychologists to be increasingly assertive about the need to recognize their particular function, status and clinical aspirations. Such aspirations were then furthered by the way in which child guidance became part of the welfare state. But just as matters seemed to be moving strongly in its direction the profession suffered a crisis of confidence with some leading mem-bers questioning the very basis of the child guidance project, hardly a stirring endorsement of what the latter sought to achieve or psychology's part in it.

Nor was child guidance psychiatry without its internal tensions. At least at the outset many leading child guidance psychiatrists publicly and routinely denied that psychoanalysis, or anything else which might probe too deeply into the child's mind to its almost certain detriment, was employed. In its place there was Moodie's 'commonsense conversation'. This, though, does not tell the whole story since even in the interwar era there is evidence that new approaches, if not strictly psychoanalytic then not far from it, were engaging individuals such as Bowlby. In turn this reminds us of the point noted above, the different approaches adopted by different clinics. In short there was no one psychiatric approach and this situ-ation continued into the post-war era, with some seeing child guidance as a form of social medicine while others began to seriously adopt a psychoanalytic stance. More fundamentally, even, there emerged a widespread questioning in psychiat-ric circles of the very expression 'child guidance', with 'child psychiatry' becoming the preferred alternative. Outside of the clinic, and in addition to the lack of suit-ably trained personnel, the way in which child guidance was integrated with the welfare state did not aid the promotion of the medical model.

Policy Context and Outcomes

This brings us to our fifth theme, the policy context and process. One obvious, and important, way of seeing child guidance provision from the 1920s to the mid-1950s is as shifting from the third sector to, primarily, the public sector. In part this was due to the nature of Commonwealth Fund financial support which was always intended to be provided only until local sources took up the slack. Voluntarism did not entirely disappear and a body such as the NAMH had important research, organization and publication functions. So there remained a mixed economy of child guidance provision.

Nonetheless, the balance and content of this mixed economy shifted and the trend was towards local authority services. Some towns and cities, most notably London, showed an interest in child guidance from its earliest days while others, for example Birmingham, were soon to be instrumental in disseminating the message outside the capital. At national level, and crucially, as it transpired, for the future, it was the Board of Education which early on adopted a watching brief and which in the 1930s formalized the powers of LEAs to provide child guidance services. It thus became increasingly likely that the latter would be dealt with under educational rather than health reconstruction. This had been almost certainly inevitable in Scotland anyway and the example of child guidance services there influenced the way in which they were introduced into English legislation.

So throughout Great Britain it was the Education Acts of the mid-1940s which embedded child guidance as part of the emerging welfare state. There were, though, confusions and lack of clarity about how what was, at least for some, a mental health service for children sat in relation to the NHS. The Ministry of Health itself, meanwhile, showed little appetite to take over child guidance provision and in any event was struggling to provide the mental health services for which it was already responsible. And while the 1959 Mental Health Act in principle promoted the expansion of community services, of which child guidance can be seen as one, in practice funding for local authorities was slow to materialize.[7]

All this, and the restricted remit of the Underwood Committee, ensured that child guidance was by and large regarded as part of the school medical service. This too gave impetus to the claims of educational psychologists as did the more prosaic fact that they were cheaper than psychiatrists. But even so, and again suggesting a lack of commitment in a significant proportion of England and Wales, the Committee reported that around one-third of local authorities were, in 1955, without any child guidance service whatsoever. In Scotland too, notwithstanding the higher status of educational psychology and the political muscle of its allies in the educational establishment, coverage was far from uniform. And, as we saw at the beginning of this chapter, ten years after Underwood the NAMH still found reasons to criticize the distribution of services. Of course much post-war welfare provision can be viewed as underfunded, including the NHS. And as we have seen child guidance early on benefitted significantly from American philanthropy, something which was not the case with most other social services, and of itself was highly resource intensive, especially if psychiatrically led. But there is a notable difference between some of the rhetoric employed about the urgent necessity for child mental health services in the national interest – the subject of our next section – and the reality.

The Child in Society

If an underlying principle of child guidance was that maladjustment in childhood could cause wider familial and social maladjustment then it followed, and again this was part of the child guidance project, that such maladjustment was potentially highly disruptive and that it thus warranted a vigorous and interventionist preventive mental health programme. This was all the more so given the relatively significant proportion of the total child population deemed to be suffering maladjustment at any particular time. The broader context here was, in the interwar era, the strains of modernity in a world – political, social, economic and even physical – characterized by instability and problems of adjustment and the insights of social sciences such as anthropology.

The Second World War, meanwhile, seemed to provide further evidence – especially although not exclusively in the form of evacuation – of the need for welfare services such as child guidance which was duly, and consciously, built into post-war social reconstruction and so became a part of the post-war political consensus. The rationale behind this was that what pre-war and wartime experience had shown was the centrality of the family to social stability. And the basis of the stable family was an emotionally and psychologically healthy relationship between the child and its parents (and indeed between the parents). Wartime pressure for child guidance came from a wide range of bodies – official and unofficial, professional and lay – and not just from its practitioners or existing proponents. The rhetoric of British social reconstruction, in an era of increasing international tension ultimately resulting in the Cold War, can be seen seeking a 'third way' – the phrase was not the invention of the late twentieth century – between communism and unbridled capitalism. In the same way, parents had to find, or be helped to find by suitably trained professionals, a middle ground between authoritarianism and licence.

And as we have seen, child guidance was not the provenance of any one political party. It was promoted by the Labour Party in the late 1930s, put into educational reconstruction at the behest of the Conservative R. A. Butler and in an Act supported more or less across the political spectrum. And whatever differences they have had over policy detail the major parties agreed that education was responsible not just for learning in the conventional sense but also for the acquisition of the characteristics of a good citizen. The child guidance argument was, of course, that such acquisition could only be realized by those in good mental health. Considerable responsibility was thus placed on children or, in reality, their parents albeit with the support, supervision and if necessary intervention of social services such as child guidance. Individual parents might be poor at parenting but could be re-educated, not least through child guidance services, since a bad parent was better than no parent. And, unsurprisingly given the gender relations of the time, much of this attention to parents in fact meant attention to mothers, although as we saw in the last chapter, some practition- ers were beginning look to fathers as well. Again this made a certain amount of sense given that, for instance, a breakdown in the relationship between husband and wife would, it was felt, impact on the child who would then present symp- toms at the child guidance clinic.

Child guidance can thus be seen, at least at a broader rhetorical level, as both part of and an agent for the promotion of consensus, moderation, stability, integration and adjustment, all of which were necessary for social progress in a liberal democratic society. As we saw in chapter 1, American child guidance had its origins in American Progressivism and it is not too much to argue that, post- 1945, British child guidance was a constituent of that very British form of social democracy which encompassed both major political parties. But as noted in the preceding section the extent to which such a liberal democratic or even social democratic society actually invested in, or was in the last resort committed to, child guidance is more open to question.

The Balance Sheet

In view of the above, what conclusions can be drawn from the history of British child guidance in its first three decades? To begin with, it seems likely that some children and possibly some parents attending child guidance clinics would have in some way benefitted from the experience. And while most of the patients were suffering from problems obviously distressing to themselves and their families – two of the commonest causes for referral, bed-wetting and stammering, being cases in point – in most instances these were relatively easy to resolve relatively quickly. Those with more substantial issues – and some of the clinical and social work notes examined for this volume do reveal extremely disturbing circum- stances – would have benefitted too if only in the sense that attention was drawn to them. For such reasons alone child guidance may have done a certain amount of good in individual cases and at some clinics former patients would return in later life to express gratitude for their experiences there.[8] Child guidance was, fur- thermore, crucial in highlighting the need for a greater focus on the individual child's emotional development and mental well-being and the need to view and understand these sympathetically, ideally in a family context – the shift, noted by Hendrick and cited in the introductory chapter, from bodies to minds. Finally under this point, and the gaps in their medical and psychological knowledge notwithstanding, it seems that practitioners generally acted out of concern for their child patients and sought to do their best for them, albeit that some interventions were in fact for the most part of the traditional social work type which could have been carried out without any child guidance intervention.

So far, so positive. But a more critical assessment is also required. For one thing, it was difficult to quantify the results and outcomes of child guidance interventions or to assess whether the former would have happened without the latter (and at less cost in time and resources). In turn this pointed to an even more fundamental problem, namely what was seen as constituting maladjustment. Despite valiant efforts by a number of psychiatrists in particular at the end of the period covered by this volume this issue remained problematic. That this was acknowledged to be so does not get around the problem nor did it stop the labelling of children whose behaviours in other social, cultural or historical circumstances might have been seen as acceptable or, in a favourite child guidance word, normal. Of course it is undeniable that normative judgements can and do intrude in all historical periods when discussing, in particular, mental states and their treatment. As Rose suggests, 'at any time and place, human discontents are inescapably shaped, moulded, given expression, judged and responded to in terms of certain languages of description and explanation, articulated by experts and authorities, leading to specific styles and forms of intervention'.[9]

Nonetheless, while some children were certainly helped by child guidance others were stigmatized since, for example, it was often known in the school why a child was absent from class and, more generally, this was an age which was not always very enlightened about mental health issues.[10] American scholars, meanwhile, have pointed to the development of services such as child guidance as contributing to the devaluing of motherhood and its reframing as 'pathological'. Motherhood too, it is argued, came under child guidance scrutiny and we have come across similar phenomena in Britain.[11] More generally, child guidance's relentless message of childhood as a 'dangerous age' almost certainly contributed to parental, and especially maternal, anxieties such as that of our fictional character, Ann, encountered in the introductory chapter.

And of course if defining and classifying maladjustment was problematic, so too and partly in consequence was formulating its treatment. As noted throughout this volume, practice varied between clinics and within and between professions, even in the same city. A child referred to Notre Dame Clinic in Glasgow would have a different experience from another seen at its local authority equivalent. At the former the full medically led team would be encountered.

At the latter psychologists would do the vast bulk of the work including the home visits undertaken at Notre Dame by a PSW. While welfare provision in Britain, even after 1945, retained in some fields strong local and regional differences, child guidance was undoubtedly at the disaggregated and diverse end of the spectrum. Although this allowed for intellectual and practical innovation and experiment, by the same token it also suggests a lack of clarity about what child guidance was about, how it reached its clinical and social work conclusions and how it went about treating the child patient.

Another problematic area lies in child guidance's focus on family relationships to the exclusion of material circumstances. On one level stressing the relationship between father and mother, and parents and child, was important given the significance of these relationships as to how families function. And it is also the case that mental health problems can occur in any social class, as Priscilla Norman's memoir attests. Nonetheless the conscious and deliberate neglect of the socio-economic environment undoubtedly distorted what child guidance sought to do and how social work especially saw itself and its function.[12] It seems perverse, for example, to attribute maladjustment and lack of integration to the strains of modernity while neglecting the material, psychological and moral strains of unemployment and deprivation. Post-war child guidance may have bought into the then common idea that the welfare state would ultimately provide a minimum standard of subsistence which would obviate the need for attention to the child's material environment. But the issue goes deeper than that since the emphasis on the family's emotional landscape was a founding child guidance principle.

And the issue of origins raises a further point. Child guidance would have probably developed without the intervention of American philanthropy but certainly not at the same pace nor necessarily in the same form – for better or worse. The Commonwealth Fund was keen to promote the medical model it supported in its home territory and was prepared to devote not inconsiderable resources to doing so. If in its early years British child guidance was reluctant to adopt practices much more common in the US and certainly more psychiatrically radical – notably psychoanalysis – nonetheless American influence is hard to deny and especially with respect to the psychiatrist's leading role. This led to endless and probably fruitless professional rivalries, resentments and turf wars. Again there can be seen to be positive dimensions to such professional competition in that it can be argued that the possibilities opened up by child guidance encouraged psychology to professionalize and both occupations to pay more attention to training as well as intellectually justifying their respective positions. The shifting boundaries noted above can also be seen in this light as well as being part of a more general phenomenon within welfare provision. But there is a further ironic twist here in that throughout the period under discussion there were always too few adequately trained psychiatrists. Such as there were, like their fellow child guidance practitioners to varying degrees, were ultimately unclear about what child guidance was all about in the first place.

It is here instructive to look in particular at a leading critic of child guidance from the late 1950s, the eminent social scientist Barbara Wootton. Discussing psychiatric social work, Wootton quoted a speech by Mildred Scoville which had asserted that 'all social casework has a psychological or mental hygiene aspect'. Wootton countered that while this had been widely accepted and had its positive aspects nonetheless there had been erected a 'fantastically pretentious façade'. The latter had disproportionately emphasized some aspects of social work while neglecting other equally useful and valid dimensions. In reality, furthermore, much contemporary social work employed methods little different from those of preceding eras and it is instructive to read these comments in the light of the issues raised in chapters 2 and 4. Wootton also had insightful points to make about child guidance itself. Child guidance clinics, she suggested, were an example of the principle 'that it is easier to create a new institution than to modify an existing one', by which she meant the education system. Clinics were actually disorientating for children as within them there was a permissive attitude very different from that in schools. This led to confusion in the child's mind and it was consequently difficult to see how the patient could 'acquire the integrated personality and outlook which is generally regarded as so vital an element in mental health'. There was a further, more fundamental, problem in that at least in part the 'prevailing emphasis upon the medical element in anti-social behaviour must be seen as an extension of the unique prestige enjoyed today by the medical profession'. One of the most significant outcomes of this, Wootton argued, was that 'the growing prestige associated with the practice of medicine in general and psychiatry in particular' had been 'a shifting of the boundary between medical and moral problems'. The confusion of medicine and morality was to the detriment of the former and inserted science into areas where moral judgements should predominate. Wootton also made the more general point that one of the consequences of psychiatry's influence was the 'tendency to blame individuals rather than their socio-economic circumstances for their problems'.[13]

Wootton was thus attacking child guidance, or at least the medical model, on some of its most cherished beliefs – the need for specialist clinics, its scientific basis and rejection of moral causes, its creation of integrated personalities, its specially trained social workers and the dominance of psychiatry. She was also questioning the need for its very existence, its neglect of socio-economic factors and its medicalizing of childhood behavioural problems. It is not necessary to accept all aspects of Wootton's critique – her separation of value judgements and science was very much of its time – but her trenchant comments, from a well-informed social scientist, further illuminate flaws and shortcomings in child guidance thought and practice.

The late 1950s saw child guidance under attack from a range of sources. As noted in the opening chapter the epidemiologist Jerry Morris expressed the view, a year before the publication of Wootton's book, that child guidance was 'little more than an act of faith' – a pithy summary of her analysis. In medicine, medical science and perhaps especially in medical practice, acts of faith have their part to play. If listening to and comforting an unhappy child to his or her palpable emotional benefit is based on, for example, a misguided notion of the causes of that child's unhappiness then so be it. To put it another way, we can become over-concerned with quantifiable outcomes and verifiable hypotheses particularly in areas such as child behaviour where social and historical constructions have such a part to play. And while child guidance services were eventually to disappear as psychological and social theory and practice changed some of the issues child guidance embraced remain, as current (2012) government proposals for parenting classes attest.[14] But having said that, in the last resort child guidance erred too much on the side of supposition and ideas which were normative rather than clinical, absorbed resources which might more usefully have been employed elsewhere, rejected important factors in the understanding of maladjustment and promoted too many cul-de-sacs in diagnosis and treatment. As implied at the beginning of this volume, Morris's judgement is thus harsh but on balance fair.

APPENDIX 1

Table A.1: Classification of patients at the Notre Dame Child Guidance Clinic

	Closed cases		Open cases	
	As referred	As diagnosed	As referred	As diagnosed
1. Disorders of personality. These consisted of disorders of mood – lability, depression, anxiety, hypochondriasis, or apathy – feelings of inferiority, rejection, or insecurity, and the shy, shut-in, seclusive, brooding or dreamy personality.	6%	28%	2%	54%
2. Behaviour disorders. Unmanageableness at home or school, stealing, impulsive behaviour, temper tantrums, lying, destructiveness, wandering, bullying, sadism, truanting and sex misdemeanours, in that order of frequency.	40%	6%	64%	2%
3. Habit disorders. Speech-defects, enuresis and food fads.	19%	6%	7.2%	2%
4. Glycopenic disorders. Disorders dependent on carbo-hydrate deficiency, such as insomnia, night-terrors and stealing.	-	-	-	10%
5. Psychoneuroses. Conversion hysteria, anxiety states and phobias made up this group in equal numbers.	5%	3%	7.2%	15%
6. Psychoses. Schizophrenia, manic depressive psychoses.	-	-	-	2%
7. Epilepsy	1%	2%	2%	2%
8. Mental deficiency. The dull and backward group – but such intellectual retardation was accompanied by personality, behaviour or habit disorders.	29%	18%	14.8%	8%
9. Mental disorder, occurring with and probably dependent on some physical disease. Congential lues, nutritional and developmental defects, intoxication from focal infection, post-encephalitis, rickets, hypopituitarism, chronic cardiac and respiratory disease, in the above order of frequency, made up this group.	4.4%	22%	4.4%	36%

Source: Archives, Mitchell Library Glasgow, D-TC 7/7/13, Notre Dame Child Guidance Clinic, *Notre Dame Child Guidance Clinic: Annual Report, 1933–34* (Glasgow: Notre Dame Child Guidance Clinic, [1934]).

APPENDIX 2

Cameron's classification system, 1955[1]

Three underlying assumptions:

1. The child is a maturing, developing organism.
2. This maturation and development is taking place in relation to an external (and internal) environment, to which the child is reacting and adapting – some of these reactions and adaptations becoming established in the child.
3. The child is an individual pursuing his/her own aims and purposes.

Four questions to be posed when the child shows disturbance:

1. Is the child potentially normal and capable of meeting the demands of the environment?
2. Is the environment meeting the needs of the child?
3. Is the environment making normal demands on the child?
4. How is this particular individual child in all his/her complexity as a human being meeting his/her situation?

Developmental categories:

1. Physiological maturity or development.
2. Physical handicapping or ill health.
3. Intellectual status.
4. Intellectual handicapping – specific and general.
5. Emotional maturity.[2]
6. Variant of personality type.

Reactive categories, i.e. reaction to his/her environment by the child:

1. Primary habit disturbance – of eating, elimination, sleeping.
2. Secondary habit disorders – gratification habits, tension habits.

3. Motor symptomatology – speech disturbance.
4. Disturbance in personal relationships – dependence, jealousy reactions.
5. Conduct disorders – delinquency.
6. Educational or work disturbance.

Individual characteristics and responses:

1. Psychic symptoms – e.g. fears, phobias, minor obsessional traits.
2. Somatic symptoms – e.g. headaches, stomach aches.
3. Psychoneurotic syndrome – anxiety state, obsessional neurosis, hysteria, etc.
4. Psychosomatic syndrome – asthma, eczema, etc.
5. Organic syndrome – diffuse cerebral damage from any cause, showing symptoms.
6. Psychotic syndrome – schizophrenia, depression, etc.
7. Attack disorder.

NOTES

Introduction: 'An Enigma to their Parents'

1. N. H. M. Burke and E. Miller, 'Child Mental Hygiene – Its History, Methods and Problems', *British Journal of Medical Psychology*, 9:3 (1929), pp. 218–42, on p. 218.
2. E. Miller, 'The Difficult Child: A Medical, Psychological and Sociological Problem', *Mother and Child*, 1:5 (1930), pp. 162–7, on p. 162.
3. *Glasgow Observer* (10 October 1931), p. 3.
4. D. R. MacCalman, 'The Management of the Difficult Child', *Journal of the Royal Institute of Public Health and Hygiene*, 1:2 (1937), pp. 93–6, on p. 95.
5. Ministry of Education, *Report of the Committee on Maladjusted Children* (London: HMSO, 1955), pp. 3, 4.
6. 'Symposium on Operational Health in the National Health Service', *Proceedings of the Royal Society of Medicine: Section of Epidemiology and Preventive Medicine*, 51:3 (1958), pp. 139–45, on p. 139.
7. H. Hendrick, *Child Welfare: Historical Dimensions, Contemporary Debate* (Bristol: The Policy Press, 2003), ch. 1, pp. 138–9.
8. N. Rose, *The Psychological Complex: Psychology, Politics and Society in England, 1869–1939* (London: Routledge and Kegan Paul, 1985), pp. 203, 202.
9. N. Rose, 'Disorders Without Borders? The Expanding Scope of Psychiatric Practice', *BioSocieties*, 1:4 (2006), pp. 465–84, on p. 472.
10. D. Armstrong, 'The Rise of Surveillance Medicine', *Sociology of Health and Illness*, 17:3 (1995), pp. 393–404, on pp. 393, 395, 396.
11. On the Commonwealth Fund, see A. McG. Harvey and S. L. Abrams, *'For the Welfare of Mankind': The Commonwealth Fund and American Medicine* (Baltimore, MD: Johns Hopkins University Press, 1986).
12. Ministry of Health, *Report of the Committee on Social Workers in the Mental Health Services: Cmd.8260* (London: HMSO, 1951), p. 11.
13. Ministry of Education, *Report of the Committee on Maladjusted Children*, p. 13.
14. For the historiography see J. Stewart, 'The Scientific Claims of British Child Guidance, 1918–45', *British Journal for the History of Science*, 42:3 (2009), pp. 407–32.
15. A. Wooldridge, *Measuring the Mind: Education and Psychology in England, c. 1860–c. 1990* (Cambridge: Cambridge University Press, 1994).
16. M. Thomson, *Psychological Subjects: Identity, Culture, and Health in Twentieth Century Britain* (Oxford: Oxford University Press, 2006), p. 117.

17. D. Thom, 'Wishes, Anxiety, Play, and Gestures: Child Guidance in Inter-War England', in R. Cooter (ed.), *In the Name of the Child: Health and Welfare, 1880–1940* (London: Routledge, 1992), pp. 200–19.

18. S. Hayes, 'Rabbits and Rebels: The Medicalisation of Maladjusted Children in Mid-Twentieth Century Britain', in M. Jackson (ed.), *Health and the Modern Home* (London: Routledge, 2007), pp. 128–52.

19. O. Sampson, *Child Guidance: Its History, Provenance and Future* (London: British Psychological Society, 1980); R. S. Addis, *History of the Child Guidance Movement* (London: The National Association for Mental Health, 1952); J. Bowlby, 'A Historical Perspective on Child Guidance', *Child Guidance Trust: Newsletter No. 3* (June 1987), pp. 1–2.

20. R. Cooter, 'In the Name of the Child Beyond', in M. Gijswit-Hofstra and H. Marland (eds), *Cultures of Child Health in Britain and the Netherlands in the Twentieth Century* (Amsterdam: Rodopi, 2003), pp. 287–96, on pp. 288–9.

21. K. W. Jones, *Taming the Troublesome Child: American Families, Child Guidance, and the Limits of Psychiatric Authority* (Cambridge, MA: Harvard University Press, 1999), p. 9 and for references to other scholars of American child guidance.

22. M. Thomson, 'Mental Hygiene as an International Movement', in P. Weindling (ed.) *International Health Organisations and Movements* (Cambridge: Cambridge University Press, 1995), pp. 283–304.

23. D. K. Henderson, 'Mental Hygiene', *Glasgow Medical Journal*, 99:6 (1923), pp. 338–59, on p. 338.

24. 'Mental Health and Social Problems: Conference in London', *British Medical Journal*, 2 (1929), p. 863 (herafter *BMJ*).

25. W. Moodie, *Child Guidance by Team Work* (London: Child Guidance Council, 1931), p. 7.

26. N. Rose, *Governing the Soul: The Shaping of the Private Self* (London: Routledge, 1989), p. 129.

27. 'Canonbury Tower and the London Child Guidance Clinic', *Journal of the London Society*, 208 (June 1935), p. 95. A copy of this article can be found at the London Metropolitan Archives (hereafter, LMA), E/NOR/Y/12.

28. W. Graebner, 'The Unstable World of Benjamin Spock: Social Engineering in a Democratic Culture, 1917–1950', *Journal of American History*, 67:3 (1980), pp. 612–29, on p. 614.

29. S. van Dijken, R. van der Veer, M. van Ijzendoorn and H.-J. Kuipers, 'Bowlby before Bowlby: The Sources of an Intellectual Departure in Psychoanalysis and Psychology', *Journal of the History of the Behavioural Sciences*, 34:3 (1998), pp. 247–69, on pp. 253–6.

30. E. F. M. Durbin and J. Bowlby, *Personal Aggressiveness and War* (London: Kegan Paul, Trench, Trubner and Co., 1939), pp. 98–9.

31. Liverpool Local Record Office (hereafter, LRO), HQ360.5 QUA, Dr M. Barton Hall, 'Mental Hygiene in Liverpool', *Liverpool Quarterly*, 1:6 (1933), pp. 3–11, on pp. 9–10.

32. Thomson, *Psychological Subjects*, p. 61.

33. Jones, *Taming the Troublesome Child*, pp. 52–3.

34. C. E. Rosenberg, 'Holism in Twentieth Century Medicine', in C. Lawrence and G. Weisz (eds), *Greater Than the Parts: Holism in Biomedicine, 1920–1950* (New York: Oxford University Press, 1998), pp. 335–55, on p. 345.

35. M. Gelder, 'Adolf Meyer and his Influence on British Psychiatry', in G. E. Berrios and H. Freeman (eds), *150 Years of British Psychiatry* (London: Athlone, 1991), pp. 419–35.

36. See D. K. Henderson and R. D. Gillespie, *A Textbook of Psychiatry for Students and Practitioners*, 7th edn (London: Oxford University Press, 1950).

37. Dr R. H. Crowley, *Child Guidance Clinics, with Special Reference to American Experience* (London: Child Guidance Council, 1928), pp. 3–4.

38. For a recent account of the role of professionals such as psychiatrists and psychologists in reshaping American motherhood in the period after 1918, and especially their role in blaming mothers for their children's perceived shortcomings, see R. J. Plant, *Mom: The Transformation of Motherhood in Modern America* (Chicago, IL: University of Chicago Press, 2010).

39. University of Liverpool, Archives and Special Collections (hereafter, UoL), EX 65:33, The Liverpool Child Guidance Council, *Report for the Year 1933* (Liverpool: The Liverpool Child Guidance Council, [1934]), p. 25.

40. *Mental Welfare*, 17:1(1936), p. 20.

41. Rockefeller Archive Center, New York, Commonwealth Fund Archives (hereafter, CF), series 16, English Mental Hygiene Program, box 3, folder 33, letter, 24 March 1939, Miss Goddard, Child Guidance Council, to Miss Scoville, Commonwealth Fund.

42. *Mental Welfare*, 17:4 (1936), p. 116.

43. LMA, 22.06 LCC, Report of the Special Services Sub-Committee of the Education Committee, 14 February and 14 and 16 March 1938.

44. C. McCallum, 'Nerston Residential Clinic: An Experiment in Child Guidance', in W. Boyd (ed.), *Evacuation in Scotland: A Record of Events and Experiments* (Bickley: University of London Press, 1944), pp. 170–91.

45. The Scottish Women's Group on Public Welfare, *Our Scottish Towns: Evacuation and the Social Future* (Edinburgh: The Scottish Women's Group on Public Welfare, 1944), pp. 20, 42.

46. J. Nuttall, '"Psychological Socialist"; "Militant Moderate": Evan Durbin and the Politics of Synthesis', *Labour History Review*, 68:2 (2003), pp. 235–52, on pp. 242, 245.

47. C. Hurl, 'Urine Trouble: A Social History of Bedwetting and its Regulation', *History of the Human Sciences*, 24:2 (2011), pp. 48–64, on p. 51.

48. J. Stewart, 'Child Guidance in Scotland 1918–55: Psychiatry versus Psychology?', *History and Philosophy of Psychology*, 12:2 (2010), pp. 26–36; L. Paterson, *Scottish Education in the Twentieth Century* (Edinburgh: Edinburgh University Press, 2003), pp. 47–8.

49. Glasgow University Archives and Business Records Centre (hereafter, GUAB), DC 130/1/1, typescript autobiography of William Boyd [*c.* 1946], p. 342.

50. Archives, the Wellcome Library, London (hereafter, Wellcome), Papers of Robina Addis (hereafter, Addis Papers), PP/ADD/C.3/6, 'Mental Health in Childhood', summary of a speech given by E.A. Hamilton-Pearson, Senior Physician to the Children's Department of the Institute of Medical Psychology, April 1932.

51. A. Freud, 'The Theory of Children's Analysis', in A. Freud, *The Psycho-Analytical Treatment of Children: Technical Lectures and Essays* (London: Imago, 1946), pp. 55–64.

52. M. Klein, *The Psychoanalysis of Children* (London: The Hogarth Press, 1932), p. 119.

53. Wellcome, Addis Papers, PP/ADD/C.3/1, typescript 'Survey of the Present Position in Regard to the Work of the Clinic', [*c.* 1930], p. 4.

54. Thomson, *Psychological Subjects*, p. 243.

55. R. Gordon, 'The Dangerous Age of Childhood', *Mother and Child*, 9:3 (1938), pp. 80–5, on p. 84.

56. M. Jones, *Holding On* (London: Quartet Books, 1973), p. 47.

1 Child Guidance Comes to Britain

1. UoL, Papers of Sir Cyril Burt (hereafter, Burt Papers), D.191/20/1/1, The Child Guidance Council, *The Child Guidance Council* (London: The Child Guidance Council, [1929]), pp. 6–7.
2. E. M. Nevill, 'The Care of Problem Children in America', *Child Life*, new series, no. 135 (October 1925), pp. 89–90, on p. 89.
3. The following passages draw on Jones, *Taming the Troublesome Child*, ch. 2.
4. Ibid., p. 49.
5. Ibid., p. 52.
6. A. Meyer, *The Collected Papers of Adolf Meyer: Volume 4, Mental Hygiene*, ed. E. Winters (Baltimore, MD: Johns Hopkins Press, 1952), p. 258.
7. For contemporary accounts see H. L. Witmer, 'By Way of Introduction', *Smith College Studies in Social Work*, 1:1 (1930), pp. 1–5; L. M. French, *Psychiatric Social Work* (New York: The Commonwealth Fund, 1940), ch. 2; and S. H. Swift, *Training in Psychiatric Social Work at the Institute for Child Guidance, 1927–1933* (New York: The Commonwealth Fund, 1934).
8. Jones, *Taming the Troublesome Child*, p. 60.
9. D. T. Rodgers, *Atlantic Crossings: Social Politics in a Progressive Age* (Cambridge, MA: Harvard University Press, 1998), pp. 2, 3, 5.
10. N. Bakker, 'Child Guidance and Mental Health in the Netherlands', *Paedagogica Historica*, 42:6 (2006), pp. 769–91, on p. 783.
11. N. Bakker, 'Health and the Medicalisation of Advice to Parents in the Netherlands, 1890–1950', in M. Gijswijt-Hofstra and H. Marland (eds), *Cultures of Child Health in Britain and the Netherlands in the Twentieth Century* (Amsterdam: Rodopi, 2003), pp. 127–48, on p. 129 and throughout.
12. K. Ludvigsen and Å. A. Seip, 'The Establishing of Norwegian Child Psychiatry: Ideas, Pioneers, and Institutions', *History of Psychiatry*, 20:1 (2009), pp. 5–26.
13. C. L. C. Burns, 'Child Guidance on the Continent', *British Journal of Educational Psychology*, 3:3 (1933), pp. 251–67.
14. Jewish Health Organisation of Great Britain, *The East London Child Guidance Clinic: Honorary Director's Report, 1927–1932* (London: Jewish Health Organisation of Great Britain, 1933), p. 5.
15. Hendrick, *Child Welfare*, pp. 21–3.
16. For the origins and creation of the Commonwealth Fund and its subsequent history, see The Commonwealth Fund, *Historical Sketch, 1918–1962* (New York: The Commonwealth Fund, 1963); and, for its impact on American medicine, Harvey and Abrams, 'For the Welfare of Mankind'.
17. *ODNB*.
18. 'B. C. Smith 1877–1952', *Who Was Who in America: Volume 3* (Chicago, IL: Marquis Who's Who Inc., 1974).
19. The Commonwealth Fund, *Historical Sketch*, appendix C.
20. E. S. Rosenberg, 'Missions to the World: American Philanthropy Abroad', in L. J. Friedman and M. D. McGarvie (eds), *Charity, Philanthropy, and Civility in American History* (Cambridge: Cambridge University Press, 2003), pp. 241–58, on p. 242 and throughout.
21. D. C. Hammack, 'Failure and Resilience: Pushing the Limits in Depression and Wartime', in Friedman and McGarvie (eds), *Charity, Philanthropy, and Civility in American History*, pp. 263–80, on p. 274.
22. E. Macadam, *The New Philanthropy: A Study in the Relations between the Statutory and Voluntary Social Services* (London: George Allen and Unwin, 1934), p. 124.

23. Wellcome, PSY/BPS/1/2/1, BPS, Committee for Research in Education, 'Annual Report for 1928–9', pp. 1–2; and BPS, Education Section, 'Annual Report, 1929–30', p. 1.
24. H. V. Dicks, *Fifty Years of the Tavistock Clinic* (London: Routledge and Kegan Paul, 1970), pp. 1–2.
25. LMA, LCC EO/WEL/1/61, *The Institute of Medical Psychology (The Tavistock Clinic), Report for the Period 1st January to 31st December 1931* (London: The Institute of Medical Psychology, 1932), pp. 3–4.
26. For brief histories of this clinic see Jewish Health Organisation of Great Britain, *The East London Child Guidance Clinic* and Burke and Miller, 'Child Mental Hygiene'.
27. The Commonwealth Fund, *Historical Sketch*, pp. 28–9.
28. The National Archives, London (hereafter, TNA), ED 50/48, memorandum 'Precis of negotiations with the Commonwealth Fund in regard to the proposed establishment of a Child Guidance Demonstration Clinic in England', [spring 1927]; Wellcome, Addis Papers, PP/ADD/K.2/3, Memorandum, 'History of Child Guidance Council and London Child Guidance Clinic', appended to letter, March 1938, to Dr J. M. Mackintosh, Department of Health for Scotland.
29. CF, series 2, Administration Files, box 24, folder 204, memorandum, 5 April 1926, Barry Smith to Edward Harkness.
30. CF, series 16, English Mental Hygiene Program, box 10, folder 107, letter, 24 April 1926, President of the American Association of Hospital Social Workers: Section on Psychiatric Social Work, to Scoville.
31. CF, series 16, English Mental Hygiene Program, box 10, folder 107, letter, 4 June 1926, Scoville to Evelyn Fox.
32. CF, series 16, English Mental Hygiene Program, box 10, folder 107, memorandum, 27 July 1926, Scoville to Smith.
33. CF, series 2, Administration Files, box 24, folder 204, memorandum, 19 July 1926, Smith to Harkness.
34. Wellcome, Addis Papers, PP/ADD/K.2/3, Memorandum, 'History of Child Guidance Council and London Child Guidance Clinic', appended to letter, March 1938, to Dr J. M. Mackintosh, Department of Health for Scotland.
35. CF, series 16, English Mental Hygiene Program, box 1, folder 11, undated and unattributed memorandum, late 1920s.
36. CF, series 2, Administration Files, box 24, folder 204, [December 1926] memorandum, Commonwealth Fund to English Child Guidance Committee.
37. CF, series 2, Administration Files, box 24, folder 204, memorandum, 2 December 1926, Smith to Harkness.
38. CF, series 2, Administration Files, box 24, folder 204, memorandum, 10 February 1927, Smith to Harkness.
39. TNA, ED 50/48, letter, 28 March 1927, Evelyn Fox to Sir George Newman.
40. UoL, Burt Papers, D.191/20/1/1, The Child Guidance Council, *The Child Guidance Council* (London: The Child Guidance Council, [c. 1929]); Wellcome, Addis Papers, PP/ADD/C.3/9, Leaflet, *The Child Guidance Council*, 1929 and presumably published in London by the Council.
41. TNA, ED 50/48, Child Guidance Council, 'Report of the Sub-Committee appointed to consider the details of the proposed Demonstration Clinic, and to report to the Council on March 25th, 1927'.
42. P. Norman, *In Way of Understanding: Part of a Life – Lantern Slides in a Rough Time Sequence* (Godalming: The Foxbury Press, 1982), pp. 59, 60–1. I am grateful to Dr Mathew Thomson, University of Warwick, for alerting me to this work.

43. CF, series 31, 'Report of the General Director to the Directors of the Commonwealth Fund, June 5th 1928: Special Programs of the Fund', p. 11. These reports were internal documents which, in edited form, were the basis of the published annual reports.

44. The Commonwealth Fund, *Tenth Annual Report* (New York: The Commonwealth Fund, 1929), p. 61.

45. Ibid.

46. CF, series 31, 'Report of the General Directors to the Directors of the Commonwealth Fund, February 14th, 1929', p. 8.

47. CF, series 7, folders 51–3, data extracted from Reports of the Board of Directors for relevant years.

48. Child Guidance Council, *Report for the Year 1933* (London: The Child Guidance Council, [1934]), p. 19.

49. UoL, Burt Papers, D.191/20/1/7, 'Report Presented to the Child Guidance Council by the Signatories, Who Visited the United States to Enquire into the Working of the Child Guidance Clinics', [*c.* 1927/28], pp. 1–5.

50. UoL, Burt Papers, D.191/20/1/9, Miss St Clair Townsend, 'Report on Psychiatric Social Work', [*c.* 1927/28], pp. 1, 3.

51. LMA, 22.06, Education Committee of the London County Council, Report of the Special Services Sub-Committee, 7 May 1928; on Fairfield, the professionalization of social work and male opposition, see M. Thomson, *The Problem of Mental Deficiency: Eugenics, Democracy, and Social Policy in Britain, 1870–1959* (Oxford: Oxford University Press, 1998), pp. 165–6.

52. UoL, Burt Papers, 'Report of C. Spearman on the Clinics for Maladjusted Children in USA and Canada', [*c.* 1927/28], pp. 1, 2, 3.

53. Crowley, *Child Guidance Clinics*, pp. 4, 5–6, 8–10, 9.

54. Ibid., pp. 12–13, 11, 15, 16, 14.

55. LMA, 22.06, Education Committee of the London County Council, Report of the Special Services Sub-Committee, 7 May 1928.

56. Norman, *In Way of Understanding*, pp. 58, 60.

57. LMA, 22.06, Education Committee of the London County Council, Report of the Special Services Sub-Committee, 25 June and 9 July 1928.

58. Board of Education, *The Health of the School Child: Annual Report of the Chief Medical Officer of the Board of Education for the Year 1927* (London: HMSO, 1928), pp. 32, 33.

59. LMA, 22.06, Education Committee of the London County Council, Report of the Joint Sub-Committee of the Establishment, Education, and Public Health Committees, 2 July 1928.

60. CF, series 16, English Mental Hygiene Program, box 19, folder 211, Reports on English students from New York School of Social Work, July 1928.

61. CF, series 16, English Mental Hygiene Program, box 21, folder 240, undated and unsigned memorandum, but either Smith or Scoville, 1928/9.

62. Thomson, *The Problem of Mental Deficiency*, p. 164.

63. CF, series 16, English Mental Hygiene Program, box 19, folder 211, 'Institute for Child Guidance, Field Work Report – New York School, Winter Quarter – March 1929'.

64. The Commonwealth Fund, *Historical Sketch*, p. 29.

65. *BMJ*, 2 (1929), p. 28.

66. LMA, 22.06, Education Committee of the London County Council, Report of the Joint Sub-Committee of the Establishment, Education, and Public Health Committees, 1 May 1929.

67. Wellcome, Bowlby Papers (hereafter, Bowlby), PP/BOW/C.5, copy of J. Bowlby, 'A Historical Perspective on Child Guidance', *Child Guidance Trust: Newsletter No. 3* (June 1987), pp. 1–2, on p. 1.

68. *BMJ*, 2 (1929), p. 158.

69. W. Moodie, 'Child Guidance', *Mental Welfare*, 10:3 (1929), pp. 98–103, on p. 100.

70. Ibid, pp. 100, 102, 98.

71. Ibid., pp. 101, 102–3.

72. M. Horn, 'Inventing the Problem Child: "At Risk" Children in the Child Guidance Movement of the 1920s and 1930s', in R. Wollons (ed.), *Children at Risk in America: History, Concepts, and Public Policy* (Albany: State University of New York Press, 1993), pp. 141–56, on pp. 145, 150.

73. CF, series 16, English Mental Hygiene Program, box 9, folder 96, 'Report on the Work of the London Child Guidance Clinic between April 1st and December 31st 1931', pp. 2–3.

74. Wellcome, Addis Papers, PP/ADD/C.3/3, *London Child Guidance Clinic, Report for the period July 29th, 1929 to December 31st, 1931* (London: London Child Guidance Clinic, [1932]), pp. 3, 21, 7, 8, 9, 10–11.

75. Thomson, *The Problem of Mental Deficiency*, p. 232.

76. CF, series 16, English Mental Hygiene Program, box 1, folder 12. Letter, 23 January 1928, The National Committee for Mental Hygiene to the Commonwealth Fund.

77. CF, series 16, box 4, folder 46, undated typescript by W. Moodie, 'The Child Guidance Council', pp. 5–6.

78. CF, series 16, box 22, folder 259, letter, 6 March 1928, Eckhard to Scoville.

79. CF, series 16, box 18, folder 190, letter, 6 December 1928, Evelyn Fox to Barry Smith.

80. CF, series 16, box 18, folder 190, letter, 20 December 1928, Barry Smith to Evelyn Fox.

81. CF, series 16, box 2, folder 16, letter, 31 January 1929, Child Guidance Council to the Commonwealth Fund.

82. Archives and Special Collections, British Library of Political and Economic Science (hereafter, BLPES), Central Filing Registry/514/1/A, letter, 31 January 1929, Child Guidance Council to William Beveridge.

83. BLPES, Central Filing Registry/514/1/A, 'Notes of an informal meeting, 13th February 1929', attended by Burt on behalf of the Child Guidance Council and various members of the LSE.

84. CF, series 16, box 7, folder 71, 'Record of Informal Meeting of Members of the Child Guidance Council, January 21st, 1931'. This meeting was chaired by Barry Smith of the Commonwealth Fund.

85. CF, series 16, box 16, folder 164, letter, 3 March 1931, William Beveridge to Barry Smith.

86. CF, series 16, box 21, folder 241, letter, 4 February 1931, Barry Smith to Mildred Scoville.

87. CF, series 16, box 16, folder 164, memorandum, 17 December 1931, Mildred Scoville to Barry Smith.

2 Professionals

1. Thomson, *Psychological Subjects*, p. 61.

2. H. Kuklick, *The Savage Within: The Social History of British Anthropology, 1885–1945* (Cambridge Cambridge University Press, 1991), Rivers quoted on p. 157, p. 136 and ch. 4;. van Dijken, et al., 'Bowlby before Bowlby', p. 249.

3. G. A. Auden, 'The Maladjusted Child', *British Journal of Educational Psychology*, 1:3 (1931), pp. 266–76, on p. 269.
4. S. C. Brown, 'The Methods of Social Case Workers', in F. C. Bartlett, M. Ginsberg, E. J. Lindgren, R. H. Thouless and E. C. Cull (eds), *The Study of Society: Methods and Problems* (London: Kegan Paul, Trench, Trubner and Co., 1939), pp. 379–401, on pp. 386–7.
5. B. Hart, 'President's Address: Psychology and Psychiatry', *Proceedings of the Royal Society of Medicine*, 25:2 (1931), pp. 188–200, on p. 199.
6. M. Thomson, 'Psychology and the "Consciousness of Modernity" in Early Twentieth Century Britain', in M. Daunton and B. Rieger (eds), *Meanings of Modernity: Britain from the Late-Victorian Era to World War II* (Oxford: Berg, 2001), pp. 97–144, on p. 100.
7. This is not to suggest this phenomenon was new: see C. E. Rosenberg, 'Pathologies of Progress: The Idea of Civilization as Risk', *Bulletin of the History of Medicine*, 72:4 (1998), pp. 714–30. Interestingly, though, this article does provide evidence from the interwar and post-war eras which reinforce the argument being made here.
8. R. Overy, *The Morbid Age: Britain between the Wars* (London: Allen Lane, 2009), p. 4.
9. The following section draws and expands on Stewart, 'The Scientific Claims of British Child Guidance'.
10. S. Sturdy and R. Cooter, 'Science, Scientific Management, and the Transformation of Medicine in Britain, *c.* 1870–1950', *History of Science*, 36:4 (1998), pp. 421–66, on pp. 437, 449.
11. C. Lawrence, *Rockefeller Money, the Laboratory, and Medicine in Edinburgh, 1919–1930: New Science in an Old Country* (Rochester, NY: University of Rochester Press, 2005), pp. 17, 26.
12. G. N. Grob, *The Mad Among Us: A History of the Care of America's Mentally Ill* (New York: The Free Press, 1994), p. 130.
13. K. Angel, 'Defining Psychiatry: Aubrey Lewis's 1938 Report and the Rockefeller Foundation', in K. Angel, E. Jones and M. Neve (eds), *European Psychiatry on the Eve of War: Aubrey Lewis, the Maudsley Hospital and the Rockefeller Foundation in the 1930s, Medical History Supplement 22* (2003), pp. 39–56, on p. 46.
14. K. Jones, 'Law and Mental Health', in Berrios and Freeman (eds), *150 Years of British Psychiatry*, pp. 89–102, on pp. 96–7.
15. Hendrick, *Child Welfare*, pp. 21, 100, 4.
16. W. Moodie, *The London Child Guidance Clinic: A Survey* (London; London Child Guidance Clinic, [1935/6]), foreword.
17. J. Bowlby, 'The Influence of Early Environment of the Development of Neurosis and Neurotic Character', *International Journal of Psychoanalysis*, 21:2 (1940), pp. 154–78, on p. 155.
18. B. Hart, 'Work of a Child Guidance Clinic', *BMJ*, 2 (1931), pp. 528–30, on p. 528.
19. J. Drever and M. Drummond, *The Psychology of the Pre-School Child* (London: Partridge, 1929), pp. 182, 187.
20. W. Boyd, 'Preventive Work with Problem Children', in W. Boyd (ed.), *Towards a New Education* (London: Knopf, 1930), pp. 289–90, on p. 290.
21. GUAB, DC130/1/1, typescript autobiography of William Boyd, p. 250.
22. N. Rose, 'Engineering the Human Soul: Analyzing Psychological Expertise', *Science in Context*, 5:2 (1992), pp. 351–69, on pp. 353, 351 and throughout.
23. Swift, *Training in Psychiatric Social Work at the Institute for Child Guidance*, pp. 5–6, 9.
24. *Proceedings of the National Conference of Social Work* (Chicago, IL: University of Chicago Press, 1931), p. 398.

25. Child Guidance Council, *Report of the Inter-Clinic Conference 1935* (London: The Child Guidance Council, 1935), p. 38.
26. Child Guidance Council, *Proceedings of the Child Guidance Inter-Clinic Conference of Great Britain 1939* (London: The Child Guidance Council, 1939), pp. 98–9.
27. Obituary, 'Tilda Goldberg', *Guardian*, 10 January 2005, p. 19.
28. Moodie, *Child Guidance by Team Work*, p. 3.
29. R. G. Gordon, Foreword', in R. G. Gordon (ed.), *A Survey of Child Psychiatry* (London: Oxford University Press, 1939), pp. v–vii, on p. vi.
30. E. Lunbeck, *The Psychiatric Persuasion: Knowledge, Gender and Power in Modern America* (Princeton, NJ: Princeton University Press, 1994), p. 305.
31. Moodie to *BMJ*, 1 (1932), p. 39.
32. D. K. Henderson, 'Social Psychiatry: Being the Morison Lectures for 1931 at the Royal College of Physicians, Edinburgh: Third Lecture', *Edinburgh Medical Journal*, 38:7 (1931), pp. 414–38, on p. 421.
33. N. Burke and E. Miller, letter to *BMJ*, 1 (1930), pp. 45–6.
34. Moodie, *Child Guidance by Team Work*, pp. 1, 2–3, 5, 2, 4.
35. Sturdy and Cooter, 'Science, Scientific Management, and the Transformation of Medicine in Britain'.
36. See, for both child guidance in particular and the broader context, A. Turmel, *A Historical Sociology of Childhood* (Cambridge: Cambridge University Press, 2008), p. 173 and chs 2 and 3 throughout.
37. TNA, ED 50/48, letter, 26 March 1927, Rev. J. C. Pringle to the Board of Education.
38. The Feversham Committee, *The Voluntary Mental Health Services* (London: The Feversham Committee, 1939), p. 157.
39. D. R. MacCalman, 'The General Management of Maladjustment in Children', in R. G. Gordon (ed.), *A Survey of Child Psychiatry* (London: Oxford University Press, 1939), pp. 257–68, on pp. 260–1.
40. Wellcome, Addis Papers, PP/ADD/C.3/1, Typescript 'Survey of the Present Position in Regard to the Work of the Clinic', [c. 1935].
41. N. H. M. Burke, 'The Difficult Child: A Medical, Psychological and Sociological Problem: II, The Management of a Clinic', *Mother and Child*, 1:6 (1930), pp. 200–5, on p. 204.
42. Wellcome, MS.7913/8, E. Miller, 'The Development of Child Guidance', p. 2.
43. CF, series 16, box 22, folder 249, letter, 25 September 1930, Edward Mapother to Barry Smith.
44. Wellcome, Addis Papers, PP/ADD/C.3/5, William Moodie, 'Child Guidance and the Schools', reprinted from *Head Teachers Review*, February 1931 as a pamphlet, pp. 7–8.
45. Moodie, *The London Child Guidance Clinic: A Survey*, p. 6.
46. Wellcome, Addis Papers, PP/ADD/C.3/3, 'London Child Guidance Clinic, Report for Period July 29th, 1929, to December 31st, 1931', [c. 1932], p. 10.
47. B. Evans, et al., 'Managing the "Unmanageable": Interwar Child Psychiatry at the Maudsley Hospital, London', *History of Psychiatry*, 19:4 (2008), pp. 454–75, on pp. 464–5.
48. G. Richards, 'Britain on the Couch: The Popularization of Psychoanalysis in Britain, 1918–1940', *Science in Context*, 13:2 (2000), pp. 183–230, on pp. 187–8, 190, 191.
49. Thomson, *Psychological Subjects*, pp. 173, 195.
50. Durbin and Bowlby, *Personal Aggressiveness and War*.
51. John Rylands Library, University of Manchester: Archives and Special Collections, VCA/7/132, draft letter, Mary Burbury, to Carl Jung's Secretary, [early 1938].

52. E. Shorter, *A History of Psychiatry: From the Era of the Asylum to the Age of Prozac* (New York: John Wiley and Sons, 1997), p. 111.

53. Aspects of Meyer's thought are also dealt with in J. Stewart, '"The Dangerous Age of Childhood": Child Guidance and the "Normal" Child in Great Britain, 1920–1950', *Paedagogica Historica*, 47:6 (2011), pp. 785–803.

54. Moodie, 'Child Guidance'.

55. Moodie, *Child Guidance by Team Work*, pp. 4–5, emphasis in the original.

56. See, for example, H. L. Witmer, *Psychiatric Clinics for Children: With Special Reference to State Programs* (New York: The Commonwealth Fund, 1940), p. 9.

57. Child Guidance Council, *Report for the Year 1933*, p. 4.

58. Board of Education, *The Health of the School Child: Annual Report of the Chief Medical Officer of the Board of Education for the Year 1934* (London: HMSO, 1935), p. 118.

59. The Commonwealth Fund, *Nineteenth Annual Report* (New York: The Commonwealth Fund, 1938), pp. 32–3.

60. See, for instance, the discussion of Freud in Witmer, *Psychiatric Clinics for Children*, p. 23.

61. For the journal's origins see *British Journal of Educational Psychology*, 1:1 (1931); and Wellcome, PSY/BPS/1/3/3, 'Minutes of Meeting of Council, 9th May 1929'.

62. Child Guidance Council, *List of Recommended Books on Child Psychology, with Annotations* (London: Child Guidance Council, 1935).

63. Oxfordshire Local Studies Centre, Central Library, Oxford, P OXFO/371.26, *Scale Test for Estimating the Intelligence as Used by the City of Oxford Educational (Child Guidance) Clinic* (Oxford: Oxford Educational Supply, 1935), foreword and tests 4, 6.

64. Jewish Health Organisation of Great Britain, *The East London Child Guidance Clinic*, p. 8.

65. For Fortes, see Kuklick, *The Savage Within*, pp. 319–20.

66. M. Fortes, 'The Difficult Child: A Medical, Psychological and Sociological Problem. IV Education and Endowment of the Difficult Child', *Mother and Child*, 1:8 (1930), pp. 296–9.

67. The Child Guidance Council, *Report of the Inter-Clinic Conference 1935*, pp. 50–1.

68. M. Collins and J. Drever, *Psychology and Practical Life* (London: University of London Press, 1936), pp. 276, 275.

69. GUAB, DC130/1/1, typescript autobiography of William Boyd, pp. 248–50, 342.

70. Glasgow University Settlement, *Social Services for Children and Young People: Glasgow 1936–37* (Glasgow: Glasgow University Settlement, 1937), p. 24.

71. TNA, ED 50/274, Board Memorandum, M481/139, 'Child Guidance – General', 1943.

72. Wooldridge, *Measuring the Mind*, p. 149.

73. J. Hall, 'The Emergence of Clinical Psychology in Britain from 1943 to 1958 Part 1: Core Tasks and the Professsionalisation Process', *History and Philosophy of Psychology*, 9:1 (2007), pp. 29–55, on p. 31.

74. Thomson, *Psychological Subjects*, pp. 138–9.

75. D. Burnham, 'Selective Memory: A Note on Social Work Historiography', *British Journal of Social Work*, 41:1 (2011), pp. 5–21.

76. C. Nottingham, 'The Rise of the Insecure Professionals', *International Review of Social History*, 52:3 (2007), pp. 445–75; V. Long, '"Often There is a Good Deal to be Done, But Socially Rather than Medically": The Psychiatric Social Worker as Social Therapist, 1945–1970', *Medical History*, 55:2 (2011), pp. 223–39. For earlier and less developed versions of the argument presented in this chapter see J. Stewart, '"I Thought You Would Want to Come and See his Home ...": Child Guidance and Psychiatric Social Work in

Inter-War Britain', in M. Jackson (ed.), *Health and the Modern Home* (London: Routledge, 2007), pp. 111–27.

77. N. Timms, *Psychiatric Social Work in Great Britain, 1939–1962* (London: Routledge and Kegan Paul, 1964).
78. Ministry of Health, *Report of the Committee on Social Workers in the Mental Health Services*, p. 11.
79. BLPES, Minutes of School Committees/16/8, Mental Health Course Consultative Committee, 8 June 1934 and Central Filing Registry/514/2/D, letter, 12 September 1939, Professor Carr-Saunders to Barry Smith, Commonwealth Fund.
80. BLPES, Central Filing Registry/514/2/C, Minutes of the Consultative Committee of the Mental Health Course, 1 December 1938.
81. BLPES, Central Filing Registry/514/1/K, Richard Titmuss, Memorandum January 1959, 'Department of Social Science and Administration', p. 2. Titmuss was Chair of Social Administration at the LSE.
82. Jones, *Taming the Troublesome Child*, p. 78.
83. Burnham, 'Selective Memory', p. 14.
84. Jones, *Taming the Troublesome Child*, p. 191.
85. Modern Records Centre, University of Warwick (hereafter, MRC), MSS.378/APSW/P/2/2, The Association of Psychiatric Social Workers, 'Report for the Year 1936 (with foreword on years 1930–35)', p. 5.
86. That is, medical, psychiatric, psychological and social.
87. BLPES, Central Filing Registry/514/1/A, letter, 31 January 1929, Child Guidance Council to William Beveridge; and letter, 3 June 1929, Child Guidance Council to LSE.
88. CF, series 16, English Mental Hygiene Program, box 13, folder 140, letter, 24 April 1934, Moodie to Barry Smith, Commonwealth Fund.
89. For course tutors see materials in the series BLPES, Central Filing Registry/514/X/X.
90. M. Ashdown and S. C. Brown, *Social Service and Mental Health: An Essay on Psychiatric Social Workers* (London: Routledge and Kegan Paul, 1953).
91. CF, series 16, English Mental Hygiene Program, box 16, folder 166, Memorandum, 5 April 1934, Scoville to Barry Smith.
92. American psychiatric social work was more self-consciously 'theoretical'. See, for instance, Swift, *Training in Psychiatric Social Work*; and French, *Psychiatric Social Work*.
93. CF, series 16, English Mental Hygiene Program, box 23, folder 260, Memorandum, September 1935, Sybil Clement Brown, 'Some Impressions of Social Work in America, 1935'.
94. CF, series 16, English Mental Hygiene Program, box 13, folder 140, letter, 24 April 1934, Moodie to Scoville.
95. Brown, 'The Methods of Social Case Workers', pp. 379, 382, 384–5, 398.
96. Burnham, 'Selective Memory', p. 14.
97. Lunbeck remarks of the American situation that psychiatric social work was 'semi-professional … at best', and not least because it was undertaken by women: Lunbeck, *The Psychiatric Persuasion*, p. 44.
98. K. W. Jones, '"Mother Made Me Do It": Mother-Blaming and the Women of Child Guidance', in M. Ladd-Taylor and L. Umansky (eds), *'Bad' Mothers: The Politics of Blame in Twentieth-Century America* (New York: New York University Press, 1998), pp. 99–124, on p. 116.
99. BLPES, Minutes of School Committees/16/5 – Mental Health Course Academic Sub-Committee, Minutes of Meeting, April 21 1932, letter from National Council for Mental Hygiene.

100. BLPES, Central Filing Registry/514/2/A, letter, 14 April 1932, Smith to C. M. Lloyd.
101. BLPES, Minutes of School Committees/16/3/1 – Mental Health Course – Practical Training Conferences, Minutes 30 October 1935, 'Report on the Training at the London Child Guidance Clinic'.
102. BLPES, Central Filing Registry/514/2/B, 'Report of the Mental Health Course for the Commonwealth Fund, July 1937'.
103. BLPES, Minutes of School Committees/16/5 – Mental Health Course Academic Sub-Committee, Minutes of Meeting, 18 May 1939.
104. Brown and Ashdown, *Social Service and Mental Health*, p. 21.
105. R. Lubove, *The Professional Altruist: The Emergence of Social Work as a Career, 1880–1930* (Cambridge, MA: Harvard University Press, 1965), p. 21.
106. Jones, *Taming the Troublesome Child*, pp. 202–3.
107. R. S. Addis, 'A Statistical Study of Nocturnal Enuresis', *Archives of Diseases in Childhood*, 10 (1935), pp. 169–78.
108. Nottingham, 'The Rise of the Insecure Professionals', p. 469.

3 The Spread of Child Guidance in the 1930s

1. Birmingham City Archives (hereafter, BCA), BCC/BH 10/1/1/23, Minutes of the Hygiene Sub-Committee of the Education Committee, 10 November 1933.
2. Wellcome, MS.7913/8, E. Miller, 'The Development of Child Guidance', p. 4.
3. See C. Burt (ed.), *How the Mind Works* (London: George Allen and Unwin, 1945, 1st edn 1933).
4. Child Guidance Council, *Report for the Year 1938* (London: The Child Guidance Council, 1939), pp. 8–9.
5. P. J. Bowler, 'Experts and Publishers: Writing Popular Science in Early Twentieth-Century Britain, Writing Popular History of Science Now', *British Journal for the History of Science*, 39:2 (2006), pp. 159–87.
6. C. Urwin and E. Sharland, 'From Bodies to Minds in Childcare Literature: Advice to Parents in Inter-War Britain', in R. Cooter (ed.), *In the Name of the Child: Health and Welfare, 1880–1940* (London: Routledge, 1992), pp. 174–99, on p. 176 and throughout.
7. L. Fildes, 'Backwardness and Behaviour Problems', *Child Life*, new series, 3:2 (1937), pp. 27–9, on p. 28.
8. D. R. MacCalman, 'Disturbances of Sleep', *Child Life*, new series, 3:4 (1937), pp. 54–6, on pp. 54–5.
9. *Mother and Child*, 9:11 (1939), p. 421.
10. E. Miller, 'The Mechanism of Behaviour Disorders and Psycho-Neurosis in Children', *Mother and Child*, 3:6 (1932), pp. 203–7; and B. H. Robinson, 'The Social Approach to Problems of Child Guidance', *Mother and Child*, 3:10 (1933), pp. 353–5.
11. L. Jordanova, 'The Social Construction of Medical Knowledge', *Social History of Medicine*, 8:3 (2005), pp. 361–81, on p. 376.
12. TNA, MH 57/291, Lecture notes for training course, 1936.
13. 'Child Guidance Council', *Mother and Child*, 5:1 (1934), p. 26.
14. Child Guidance Council, *Report for the Year 1936* (London: Child Guidance Council, 1937), p. 11.
15. Labour Party Archives, People's History Museum, Manchester, LP/RD/3/7, draft document on education policy, 1934, pp. 31–2.
16. The Labour Party, *A Children's Charter* (London: The Labour Party, 1937), p. 25.

17. *BMJ*, 2 (1933), p. 1074.
18. Wellcome, PSY/BPS/1/2/2, 'British Psychological Society, Scottish Branch, Annual Report, 1935–36', p. 1.
19. E. Miller, 'Temperamental Differences in the Behaviour Disorders of Children', *British Journal of Educational Psychology*, 3:3 (1933), pp. 222–35.
20. LMA, 22.06 LCC, 'Report of the General Sub-Committee of the Education Committee, 14th September and 9th and 23rd November, 1943'.
21. The Commonwealth Fund, *Fifteenth Annual Report, 1934* (New York: The Commonwealth Fund, 1935), p. 62.
22. BCA, BCC/BH 1/1/1/32, Minutes of the Education Committee, 27 April 1934.
23. CF, series 16, English Mental Hygiene Program, box 3, folder 32, letter, 21 July 1938, Scoville to Gordon at Child Guidance Council; and box 3, folder 33, letter, 7 May 1939, MacCalman to Commonwealth Fund.
24. Child Guidance Council, *Report for the Year 1934* (London: The Child Guidance Council, 1935), p. 15.
25. Child Guidance Council, *Report for the Year 1935* (London: The Child Guidance Council, 1936), p. 11.
26. I. Grosvenor and K. Myers, 'Progressivism, Control and Correction: Local Education Authorities and Educational Policy in Twentieth Century England', *Paedagogica Historica*, 42:1, 42:2 (2006), pp. 225–47, on pp. 234, 244, 232.
27. BCA, BCC/BH 10/1/1/20, Minutes of the Hygiene Sub-Committee of the Education Committee, 4 December 1930.
28. J. T. Jones, *History of the Corporation of Birmingham, Vol. V, Part I* (Birmingham: General Purposes Committee Birmingham Corporation, 1940), p. 235.
29. Sampson, *Child Guidance: Its History, Provenance and Future*, p. 14.
30. BCA, BCC/BH 1/1/1/29, Minutes of the Education Committee, 19 December 1930. The actual financial arrangements turned out to be slightly different in terms of staff employment, but the underlying principles remained.
31. 'Child Guidance Council', *Mother and Child*, 1:11 (1931), p. 430.
32. BCA, BCC/BH 1/1/1/29, Minutes of the Education Committee, 30 October 1931; and BCC/BH 1/1/1/32, Minutes of the Education Committee, 26 October 1934.
33. TNA, ED 50/102, Board of Education: Interview Memorandum, M406/651/2, 27 July 1933. This file also includes various notes on consultations on the issue of funding before and after the Child Guidance Council visit.
34. Ibid.
35. See, for example, TNA, ED 50/48, Board Memorandum M406/641/2, August 1933.
36. TNA, ED 50/273, letter, 13 November 1935, Board of Education to Home Office.
37. Wellcome, MS.7913/9, cited in N. Gibbs, 'Developments in Child Guidance', p. 3.
38. Board of Education, *The Health of the School Child: Annual Report of the Chief Medical Officer of the Board of Education for the Year 1934* (London: HMSO, 1935), p. 118.
39. BCA, BCC/BH 1/1/1/32, Minutes of the Education Committee, 26 October 1934.
40. The information in this section has been collated from BCA, BCC/BH 1/1/1/35, Minutes of the Education Committee, 23 July 1937; BCC/BH 1/1/1/36, 'Annual Report to the City of Birmingham Education Committee of the School Medical Officer for the Year Ended 31st December, 1937', p. 30; BCC/BH 1/1/1/36, 'City of Birmingham Education Committee. Child Guidance Clinic. Report of the Medical Director, 1936–38'; and BCC/BH 1/1/1/37, 'Annual Report to the City of Birmingham Education Committee of the School Medical Officer for the Year Ended 31st December, 1938', p. 42.

41. C. Urwin, 'Margaret Lowenfeld', in C. Urwin and J. Hood-Williams (eds), *Selected Papers of Margaret Lowenfeld* (London: Free Association Books, 1988), pp. 3–139, p. 42.
42. 'Manchester Child Guidance Clinic', *Mental Welfare*, 19:1 (1938), p. 22; Central Library, Manchester: Local Studies and Archives (hereafter, Manchester), Minutes of the General Purposes Sub-Committee of the Education Committee, 16 October 1939, report 'Notes on Developments During the Period 1936–39', p. 5.
43. City and Council of Bristol, *The Health of Bristol in 1959* (Bristol: City and County of Bristol, 1960), section F, p. 3. I am grateful to Dr G. C. Gosling for obtaining a copy of this report.
44. 'Child Guidance', *Mental Welfare*, 17:4 (1936), p. 116.
45. 'Child Guidance Clinic, Sheffield', *Mental Welfare*, 18:4 (1937), p. 118.
46. LRO, H.360.5 QUA, copy of *Liverpool Quarterly*, 1:6 (1933), which includes an article, by Dr M. Barton Hall, 'Liverpool and Mental Hygiene', pp. 3–10, on p. 9.
47. UoL, EX 65:39, The Liverpool Child Guidance Council, *Report for the Year 1939* (Liverpool: The Liverpool Child Guidance Council, [*c.* 1940]), p. 11.
48. UoL, EX 65:33, The Liverpool Child Guidance Council, *Report for the Year 1933* (Liverpool: The Liverpool Child Guidance Council, [*c.* 1934]), pp. 1, 3, 9, 5.
49. LRO, 352 MIN/EDU II 1/12, Minutes of the Education Committee, 16 July 1934 and 352 MIN/EDU II 1/14, Minutes of the Education Committee, 22 May 1939.
50. UoL, EX 65:39, The Liverpool Child Guidance Council, *Report for the Year 1939*, p. 21.
51. A. C. Cameron, 'Education in the City of Oxford', in A. C. Cameron (ed.), *Oxford 1935: A Souvenir of the World Educational Conferences* (Oxford: Oxford University Press, 1935), pp. 245–54, on pp. 251–2.
52. TNA ED 50/273, Letter, 13 November 1935, Board of Education to Home Office.
53. See, for instance, Cameron, 'Education in the City of Oxford'; and E. F. Pinsent, *The Mental Health Services in Oxford City, Oxfordshire and Berkshire* (Oxford: Oxford University Press, 1937), pp. 18–23.
54. Child Guidance Council, *Report for the Year 1939* (London: The Child Guidance Council, 1940), p. 3.
55. The Feversham Committee, *The Voluntary Mental Health Services*, p. 153.
56. MRC, MSS.378/APSW/P/20/5 'List of Child Guidance Clinics Recognized by Child Guidance Council', [*c.* 1940].
57. National Library of Scotland, Manuscripts Division (hereafter, NLS), Acc.7170, box 1, folder 1, SAMW circular letter, 26 February 1931.
58. NLS, Acc.7170, box 1, folder 3, 'Minutes of Meeting Held in Glasgow on October 13th, 1934'.
59. NLS, Acc.7170, box 1, folder 1, 'Minutes of the Mental Hygiene Sub-Committee, 10th October 1934'.
60. On the merger see NLS, Acc.7170, box 1, folder 1, Minutes of the Executive Council, 19 February 1938.
61. Sister J. McCallum, et al., 'Foundations', in *The Notre Dame Centre, Freedom to Grow: Celebrating 75 Years of the Notre Dame Centre in Glasgow* (Glasgow: The Publishing Cupboard, 2007), pp. 8–21, on p. 10. I am grateful to Sister Gail Taylor, one of the authors of this chapter, for drawing it to my attention.
62. On this Clinic, see J. Stewart, '"An Enigma to their Parents": The Founding and Aims of the Notre Dame Child Guidance Clinic, Glasgow', *Innes Review*, 57:1 (2006), pp. 54–76.
63. CF, series 16, English Mental Hygiene Program, box 5, folder 56, letter, 22 April 1932, Child Guidance Council to Mildred Scoville.

64. CF, series 16, English Mental Hygiene Program, box 6, folder 58, Memorandum, 6 February 1933, Graham Taylor, Director of the Publications Department, CF, to Barry Smith and entitled 'Visit to Notre Dame Child Guidance Clinic, Glasgow'.
65. Wellcome, PSY/BPS/1/2/2, 'British Psychological Society, Scottish Branch, 'Annual Report, 1933–34', p. 1.
66. City Archives, Mitchell Library, Glasgow (hereafter, Mitchell), D-TC 7/7/13, Notre Dame Child Guidance Clinic, *Annual Report 1933–34* (Glasgow: Notre Dame Child Guidance Clinic, [1934]), p. 14.
67. Scottish Catholic Archives, Edinburgh (hereafter, SCA), DE 125/1, undated leaflet, *The Edinburgh Catholic Child Guidance Clinic*; DE 125/3, 'Edinburgh Catholic Child Guidance Clinic: Annual Report, April 1934 to April 1935', p. 3.
68. CF, series 16, English Mental Hygiene Program, box 13, folder 136, letter, 23 March 1932, William Moodie to Mildred Scoville.
69. GUAB, Notre Dame Training College, Glasgow: Minute Book, UGC 58/1/2/1, 'Report on Session 1931–32'.
70. Cited in Sister Jude, *Freedom to Grow: Sister Marie Hilda's Vision of Child Guidance* (Glasgow: John S. Burns and Sons, 1981), pp. 32–3.
71. SCA, DE 125/15, exchange of letters between Miss Lamb and Mr Weldon, St Vincent de Paul Society, May to July 1933.
72. Sister Jude, *Freedom to Grow*, p. 42.
73. Mitchell, C1/3/96a, Minutes of a Joint Meeting of the Sub-Committees on Mental Services and Teachers and Teaching, 18 May 1937.
74. SCA, DE 125/27, letter, 14 January 1935, Lady Margaret Kerr to Liverpool and District Child Guidance Council.
75. CF, series 16, English Mental Hygiene Program, box 6, folder 60, letter, 5 July 1934, Douglas MacCalman to the Child Guidance Council.
76. Sister Jude, *Freedom to Grow*, p. 33.
77. *Tablet*, 172:5:139 (1938), p. 614.
78. SCA, DE 125/27, letter, 14 January 1935, Lady Margaret Kerr to Liverpool and District Child Guidance Council.
79. SCA, DE 125/35, notes by Miss Meredith, 2 October 1934.
80. 'A Little Child Shall Lead Them', *Tablet*, 155:4:702 (1930), p. 825.
81. Stewart, '"An Enigma to their Parents"', p. 66.
82. SCA, DE 125/38, letter, 4 February 1935, Peter Mellon to Miss Meredith.
83. SCA, DE 125/31, letter, 7 July 1937, Lady Moncrieff to Lady Dalrymple.
84. Stewart, '"An Enigma to their Parents"', p. 60.
85. SCA, DE 122/2, letter, 11 February 1934, Mildred Macgown to the Archbishop of St Andrews and Edinburgh.
86. SCA, DE 125/23, letter, 26 June 1935, Lady Margaret Kerr to Miss M.G. Cowan.
87. SCA, DE 125/32, cutting from *Universe*, April 1937.
88. Cited in Sister Jude, *Freedom to Grow*, p. 1.
89. Sister Marie Hilda, *Child Guidance* (London: Catholic Truth Society, 1950), p. 6.
90. Ibid., p. 8.
91. See also Stewart, '"An Enigma to their Parents"', p. 68.
92. Sister Marie Hilda, *Child Guidance*, p. 15.
93. M. D. L. Dickson, *Child Guidance* (London: Sands and Co., 1938), pp. 151–3.
94. SCA, DE 125/35, Miss Meredith's notes of meeting with Miss Ashley, 5 November 1934.

95. D. R. MacCalman, 'The Present Status and Functions of the Child Guidance Movement in Great Britain, and its Possible Future Developments', *Journal of Mental Science*, 85 (1939), pp. 505–21, on p. 511.

96. The argument in J. Stewart, 'Child Guidance in Interwar Scotland: International Context and Domestic Concerns', *Bulletin of the History of Medicine*, 80:3 (2006), pp. 513–39 is thus significantly modified.

97. Sir A. Macgregor, *Public Health in Glasgow, 1905–1946* (Edinburgh: E. & S. Livingstone, 1967), p. 133.

98. G. Dell, 'Thirty Years of Child Guidance: The Development of the Glasgow Child Guidance Service', *Scottish Educational Research*, 1:3 (1969), pp. 32–8, on p. 33.

99. C. M. McCallum, 'Symposium on Psychologists and Psychiatrists in the Child Guidance Service: IV Child Guidance in Scotland', *British Journal of Educational Psychology*, 22:2 (1952), pp. 79–88, on p. 79 and note 1.

100. Edinburgh City Archives, 'Council Record, 1931–2', p. 33; 'Council Record, 1934–5', pp. 45–6; and, for example, SL 164/1/8, Minutes of the Education Committee, 25 March 1935, delegating Dr Sym to the General Council of the Scottish Child Guidance Council.

101. Edinburgh Corporation Education Committee, *Education Week 1936* (Edinburgh: Edinburgh Corporation, 1936), p. 172.

102. Child Guidance Council, *Report for the Year 1939*, p. 4.

103. Dundee University Archives (hereafter, DUA), RU565/1/13, Minutes of the Meeting of the St Andrews Provincial Committee for the Training of Teachers, 1 June 1932; and RU565/1/14, 'Report by the Director of Studies on the Training of Students and the Committee's Work throughout the Province during the Session 1932–33, 30th October 1933'.

104. Dundee City Archives (hereafter, DCA), Minutes of a Meeting of the Education Committee, 12 December 1933; and Minutes of a Meeting of the Education Committee, 28 April 1936.

105. DUA, RU565/1/15, 'Report of the Director on the Training of Students and the Committee's work throughout the Province during the Session 1935–36, 30th October 1936'.

106. City of Dundee, *Report of the Medical Officer of Health for the Year Ending 31st December, 1936* (Dundee: Dundee City Council, 1937), p. 12.

107. DUA, RU565/1/15, 'Report of the Director on the Training of Students and the Committee's work throughout the Province during the Session 1935–36, 30th October 1936'.

108. DUA, RU565/1/16, Report by the Director of Studies on the Training of Students and the Committee's work throughout the Province during the Session 1937–37, 30th October 1937'.

109. See Paterson, *Scottish Education in the Twentieth Century*, pp. 47–8.

110. Scottish Education Department, *Report of the Committee of Council on Education in Scotland for the Year 1938* (Edinburgh: HMSO, 1939), pp. 41–2.

111. MRC, MSS.378/APSW/P/20/5, [early 1940s], list of recognized child guidance clinics.

4 Normalcy, Happiness and Child Guidance in Practice

1. This chapter draws in part on Stewart, '"The Dangerous Age of Childhood": Child Guidance and the "Normal" Child in Great Britain, 1920–1950'.

2. The Feversham Committee, *The Voluntary Mental Health Services*, p. x.

3. CF, series 16, English Mental Hygiene Program, box 10, folder 99, cutting from *The Times*, 22 January 1937.

4. 'Discussion on the Difficult Child', *Proceedings of the Royal Society of Medicine*, 23:4 (1930), pp. 573–85, on p. 578.
5. C. L. C. Burns, 'Birmingham Child Guidance Clinic: A Review of Two Years' Work', *Mental Welfare*, 16 (1935), p. 7.
6. MacCalman, 'The Present Status and Functions of the Child Guidance Movement in Britain', p. 509.
7. Moodie, *Child Guidance by Team Work*, p. 1.
8. W. Moodie, 'Some Problems of Childhood: Methods of Treatment', *Mother and Child*, 2:7 (1931), pp. 259–61, on p. 260.
9. F. Bodman, 'Psychological Development of the Child', *Mother and Child*, 14:11 (1944), pp. 215–7, on pp. 215, 217.
10. The National Archives of Scotland (hereafter, NAS), ED 15/108, Minutes of the Thirteenth Meeting of the Scottish Advisory Council on the Treatment and Rehabilitation of Offenders, 21 September 1945, p. 2.
11. MacCalman, 'The General Management of Maladjustment in Children', pp. 265–6.
12. D. Armstrong, *A New History of Identity: A Sociology of Medical Knowledge* (Basingstoke: Palgrave, 2002), p. 102.
13. SCA, DE 125/11, letter, 1 November 1933, Miss Lamb to Mrs Kathleen Jones.
14. P. C. Shapiro, *How Child Guidance Contributes to Mental Health* (London: Child Guidance Council, 1933), p. 3.
15. Mitchell, D-TC 7/7/13, Notre Dame Child Guidance Clinic, *Notre Dame Child Guidance Clinic: Annual Report, 1933–34*, pp. 5–6, 9–11. A table showing more detail of the classification system can be found in appendix 1, p. 185.
16. BCA, BCC/BH 1/1/1/36, 'City of Birmingham Education Committee. Child Guidance Clinic. Report of the Medical Director, 1936–1938', pp. 5–7.
17. E. Miller, 'Right and Wrong', *Child Life*, 4:1 (1938), pp. 6–8, on pp. 6–7.
18. Wellcome, PP/BOW/C.3/1, undated flyer produced by the London Child Guidance Clinic.
19. Henderson and Gillespie, *A Textbook of Psychiatry for Students and Practitioners*, p. 635.
20. H. Gillespie, 'Psychiatric Problems of Children under Five Years', *Mother and Child*, 25:11 (1955), pp. 272–4, on p. 272.
21. S. Cohen, 'The Mental Hygiene Movement, the Development of Personality and the School: The Medicalization of American Education', *History of Education Quarterly*, 23:2 (1983), pp. 123–49, on p. 131.
22. C. Lane, *Shyness: How Normal Behaviour Became a Sickness* (New Haven, CT: Yale University Press, 2007), pp. 2, 14, 8.
23. Hayes, 'Rabbits and Rebels'.
24. Turmel, *A Historical Sociology of Childhood*, p. 182.
25. Rose, 'Disorders without Borders?', p. 475.
26. C. E. Rosenberg, 'Contested Boundaries: Psychiatry, Disease and Diagnosis', *Perspectives in Biology and Medicine*, 49:3 (2006), pp. 407–24, on p. 411.
27. C. E. Rosenberg, 'What is Disease? In Memory of Owsei Temkin', *Bulletin of the History of Medicine*, 77:3 (2003), pp. 491–505, on pp. 501–2.
28. P. Stearns, 'Defining Happy Childhoods: Assessing a Recent Change', *Journal of the History of Childhood and Youth*, 3:2 (2010), pp. 165–86.
29. Miss McTaggart, 'A Psychologist at the Conference', *Child Life Quarterly*, new series, 160 (1933), pp. 48–50, on p. 49.

30. C. L. C. Burns, 'What Can Local Authorities Do For the Maladjusted Child?', *Mother and Child*, 9:10 (1939),pp. 371–2, on p. 372.

31. BLPES HQ/60, William Moodie, *The Unstable Child: An Address Given for the Child Guidance Council at the Twenty-Second Annual Conference of Educational Authorities, January 1934*, reprinted from the Report of the Conference of Educational Associations.

32. MacCalman, 'The General Management of Maladjustment in Children', p. 266.

33. LRO, 352 MIN/EDU II 5/7, typescript 'The Liverpool and District Child Guidance Council and Clinic, April 4th 1938 – Report on Cases Dealt with at this Clinic during 1937', pp. 3–4.

34. D. R. MacCalman, 'Address to Mothers: Familiar Problems of Child Upbringing', *Mother and Child*, 8:3 (1937), pp. 90–1, on p. 91.

35. J. Bowlby, *Child Care and the Growth of Love* (Harmondsworth: Penguin Books, 1953), p. 1.

36. DCA, TC/SF/Ed53, 'Summary of Cases Referred to the Child Guidance Clinic During the Period from September 1st 1936 to November 30th 1940'.

37. Mitchell, D-TC, 7/7/13, Notre Dame Child Guidance Clinic, *Annual Report, 1938–9* (Glasgow: Notre Dame Child Guidance Clinic, [1939]), pp. 5, 12, 6.

38. Wellcome, Addis Papers, PP/ADD/C.3/3, London Child Guidance Clinic, *Report for the Period July 29th, 1929 to December 31st, 1931* (London: London Child Guidance Clinic, [1932]), p. 8.

39. UoL, EX 65:37, The Liverpool Child Guidance Council, *Report for the Year 1937* (Liverpool: Liverpool Child Guidance Council, [1938]), p. 14.

40. The Feversham Committee, *The Voluntary Mental Health Services*, p. 151.

41. LMA, 22.06 LCC, 'Report of the Special Services Sub-Committee, 20th March and 24th April 1933'.

42. SCA, DE 125/3, 'Edinburgh Catholic Child Guidance Clinic: Report for the Year January 1933 to December 1933', pp. 1, 2, 4.

43. Dickson, *Child Guidance*, pp. 44–58.

44. Jones, '"Mother Made Me Do It"', p. 107.

45. Wellcome, Addis Papers, PP/ADD/C.1/8 and PP/ADD/C.1/9 – these case notes have been accessed on the understanding and condition that individuals are anonymized.

46. Wellcome, Addis Papers, PP/ADD/C.1/10.

47. Bowlby, 'The Influence of Early Environment in the Development of Neurosis and Neurotic Character', pp. 164–7.

48. R. Levinson, 'Expression of the Neuroses in Childhood', *Mother and Child*, 4:9 (1933), pp. 339–41, on pp. 339–40.

49. B. H. Robinson, 'The Difficult Child: A Medical, Psychological and Sociological Problem. III. The Function of the Social Worker', *Mother and Child*, 1:7 (1930), pp. 249–52, on pp. 251–2.

50. SCA DE 125/X. Access to these case records was granted on the condition that the individual files, and the children's names, were anonymized.

51. I am grateful to Dr Hera Cook for this point and on which see H. Cook, *The Long Sexual Revolution: English Women, Sex, and Contraception, 1800–1975* (Oxford: Oxford University Press, 2004), pp. 147, 210.

52. Bowlby, 'A Historical Perspective on Child Guidance', p. 2.

53. Jones, '"Mother Made Me Do It"', pp. 114, 108, and throughout.

54. Plant, *Mom*, p. 3.

55. Moodie, *The London Child Guidance Clinic: A Survey*, p. 6.

56. BCA, BCC/BH 1/1/1/36, 'City of Birmingham Education Committee. Child Guidance Clinic. Report of the Medical Director, 1936–1938', p. 3.
57. BCA, BCC/BH 10/1/1/27, Minutes of the Hygiene Sub-Committee of the Education Committee, 7 July 1938 and 15 September 1938.
58. BCA, BC/BH 10/1/1/28, Minutes of the Hygiene Sub-Committee of the Education Committee, 11 May 1939.
59. CF, series 16, English Mental Hygiene Program, box 6, folder 58, cutting from *Liverpool Post and Mercury*, 28 January 1933.
60. Moodie, 'Some Problems of Childhood', pp. 260–1.
61. Burns, 'Birmingham Child Guidance Clinic', p. 7.
62. BCC/BH 1/1/1/36, 'City of Birmingham Education Committee. Child Guidance Clinic. Report of the Medical Director, 1936–38', p. 8.
63. Moodie, *The London Child Guidance Clinic: A Survey*, p. 7.
64. Library of the Wellcome Unit for the History of Medicine, University of Oxford, WX 28 FE5.2 Lon Guys, *Report of the Institution and Development of the Child Guidance Clinic at Guy's Hospital London, 1930–1936* (London: Guy's Hospital, [1936/7], p. 10, Table 4 – the other categories, making up to 100 per cent, were 'In Institutions' and 'Not Traced'.
65. BCA, BCC/BH 1/1/1/36, 'City of Birmingham Education Committee. Child Guidance Clinic. Report of the Medical Director, 1936–1938', p. 8.
66. C. W. Valentine, *The Difficult Child and the Problem of Discipline* (London: Methuen, 1940), pp. 35–6.
67. LMA, 22.06, LCC, 'Report of the Special Services Sub-Committee of the Education Committee, 16th March 1936'.
68. The Feversham Committee, *The Voluntary Mental Health Services*, p. 151.
69. J. Rickman, 'Preface', in J. Rickman (ed.), *On the Bringing Up of Children* (London: Paul, Trench, and Trubner, 1936), pp. 7–14, on pp. 8–10.

5 Child Guidance in Wartime

1. For the most recent analysis of evacuation see J. Welshman, *Churchill's Children: The Evacuee Experience in Wartime Britain* (Oxford: Oxford University Press, 2010).
2. TNA, ED 50/273, letter, May 1939, Board of Control to Board of Education.
3. *Mother and Child*, 10:8 (1939), p. 314.
4. Wellcome, Addis Papers, PP/ADD/H.5, Typescript, 30 September 1944, 'The Work of the Provisional National Council'. The Child Guidance Council continued to use its own name, however, even when subsumed into the Emergency Committee. The latter became, after a period as the Provisional National Council for Mental Health, the National Association for Mental Health, on the founding of which see Norman, *In the Way of Understanding*, pp. 138–9.
5. TNA, ED 50/273, letter, 16 May 1939, Mental Health Emergency Committee to Board of Education.
6. R. Titmuss, *Problems of Social Policy* (London: HMSO, 1950), pp. 102–3.
7. The Scottish Women's Group on Public Welfare, *Our Scottish Towns*, pp. 18–20.
8. W. Moodie, *The Doctor and the Difficult Child*, 2nd edn (New York: The Commonwealth Fund, 1947), p. xi.
9. Ministry of Education, *The Health of the School Child: Report of the Chief Medical Officer of the Ministry of Education for the Years 1939–1945* (London: HMSO, 1947), pp. 64, 65.

10. Durbin and Bowlby, *Personal Aggressiveness and War*; van Dijken, et al., 'Bowlby before Bowlby', p. 256, where the authors suggest that Isaacs was actively engaged in Bowlby's supervision.

11. B. Mayhew, 'Between Love and Aggression: The Politics of John Bowlby', *History of the Human Sciences*, 19:4 (2006), pp. 19–35, on p. 26.

12. Titmuss, *Problems of Social Policy*, pp. 19–20.

13. TNA, ED 50/273, 'Board of Education: Interview Memorandum: Behaviour Problems Among Evacuated Children', M481/33 (4), 30 September 1939.

14. CF, series 16, English Mental Hygiene Program, box 5, folder 48, 'Summary of John Bowlby's paper for the 1939 Inter-Clinic Conference'.

15. Mrs St Loe Strachey, *Borrowed Children: A Popular Account of Some Evacuation Problems and their Remedies* (New York: The Commonwealth Fund, 1940), p. 133. It is, of course, possible that this was Bowlby.

16. A. Freud and D. Burlingham, *Infants without Families and Reports of the Hampstead Nurseries, 1939–1945* (London: The Hogarth Press, 1974), p. 208 citing 1942 Annual Report.

17. TNA, ED 50/273, letter, 11 October 1939, Board of Education to Association of Education Committees.

18. TNA, ED 50/274, cutting from *Medical Officer*, 28 October 1939.

19. BLPES, Minutes of School Committees/16/3/1 – Mental Health Course – Practical Training Conferences, minutes 28 June 1943.

20. CF, series 31, Reports of the General Director, 'Report of the General Director to the Directors of the Commonwealth Fund, December 14th, 1939', p. 50.

21. E. H. Jones, *Margery Fry: The Essential Amateur* (York: The Ebor Press, 1966), p. 219.

22. UoL, EX 65:39, The Liverpool Child Guidance Council, *Report for the Year 1939*, pp. 13, 18.

23. John Rylands Library, University of Manchester, Medical Collection, City of Manchester Education Committee, *Annual Report of the Acting School Medical Officer, Dr J. Gilbert Woolham, 1939* (Manchester: Manchester Corporation, 1940), p. 13; and City of Manchester Education Committee, *Annual Report of the Acting School Medical Officer, Dr J. Gilbert Woolham, 1940 and 1941* (Manchester: Manchester Corporation, 1942), p. 41.

24. Mitchell, CO 1/5/3/10, Minutes of the Attendance and Administration Sub-Committee, Education Committee of the Council of Lanark, 2 November 1939, appendix 1.

25. J. Bowlby, 'Psychological Aspects', in R. Padley and M. Cole (eds), *Evacuation Survey* (London: George Routledge and Sons, 1940), pp. 186–96, on pp. 186, 195, 188.

26. McCallum, 'Nerston Residential Clinic', pp. 170–2, 189.

27. C. Burt and C. A. Simmins, 'The Cambridge Evacuation Survey', *British Journal of Educational Psychology*, 12:2 (1942), pp. 71–5, on pp. 72–3.

28. BLPES, Central Filing Registry/514/2/D, letter, 12 September 1939, Carr-Saunders to Barry Smith.

29. BLPES, Central Filing Registry/514/1/F, letter, 4 December 1940, Sybil Clement Brown to Carr-Saunders; and Minutes of School Committees/16/3/1 – Mental Health Course – Practical Training Conferences, minutes 28 November 1942; The Commonwealth Fund, *The Twenty-Fourth Annual Report of the Commonwealth Fund* (New York: The Commonwealth Fund, 1943), p. 16.

30. *London Children in War-Time Oxford: A Survey of Social and Educational Results of Evacuation* (London: Oxford University Press, 1947), preface.

31. MRC, MSS.378/APSW/P/11/1, Sybil Clement Brown, memorandum, 'Training for Psychiatric Social Work: The Mental Health Course in Wartime', [c. 1942].

32. E. Davies, 'Psychiatric Treatment for Difficult Evacuees', *National Froebel Foundation Bulletin*, 9 (1941), pp. 5–6, on p. 5.

33. J. C. Kenna, *Educational and Psychological Problems of Evacuation: An Analysis of Experience in England* (Melbourne: Australian Council for Educational Research, 1942), pp. 29–32, 40.

34. P. H. Cook, *The Theory and Technique of Child Guidance* (Melbourne: Australian Council for Educational Research/Melbourne University Press, 1944), pp. 9, 14, 26.

35. MRC, MSS.378/APSW/P/11/1, letter, 29 October 1941, American Association of Psychiatric Social Workers to Noel Hunnybun.

36. Ministry of Education, *Report of the Committee on Maladjusted Children*, p. 12.

37. Child guidance clinics and practitioners also played a part in the care of more severely disabled children, often in hostels or other institutions – see S. Wheatcroft, 'Cured by Kindness? Child Guidance Services during the Second World War', in A. Borsay and P. Dale (eds), *Disabled Children: Contested Caring, 1850–1979* (London: Pickering & Chatto, 2012), pp. 145–57.

38. 'Preface' and 'Introduction', in S. Isaacs, (ed.), *The Cambridge Evacuation Survey: A Wartime Study in Social Welfare and Education* (London: Methuen, 1941), preface, pp. v–vii, on p. vi and introduction, pp. 1–11, on p. 7.

39. 'Child Guidance in a Reception Area', in Isaacs (ed.), *The Cambridge Evacuation Survey*, pp. 109–22, on p. 111, 116–7, 118.

40. Ibid., p. 111.

41. Ibid., pp. 120, 118.

42. Ibid., p. 115, case 3.

43. F. Bodman, 'Enemy Action', in *The Future of Child Guidance in Relation to War Experience* (London: The Child Guidance Council, 1941), pp. 1–7, on pp. 1, 2, 7.

44. City and County of Bristol, *The Health of Bristol in 1959*, section F, p. 3.

45. MRC, MSS.378/APSW/P/20/5, list of child guidance clinics recognized by Child Guidance Council [c. 1940].

46. Ministry of Education, *Report of the Committee on Maladjusted Children*, p. 12.

47. McCallum, 'Symposium on Psychologists and Psychiatrists in the Child Guidance Service IV Child Guidance in Scotland', p. 80.

48. Dell, 'Thirty Years of Child Guidance: The Development of the Glasgow Child Guidance Service', p. 35.

49. SCA, DE 122/5, cutting from the *Scotsman* [c. 1942].

50. The Commonwealth Fund, *Twenty-Fifth Annual Report of the Commonwealth Fund* (New York: The Commonwealth Fund, 1944), p. 25.

51. *Mother and Child*, 13:8 (1942), pp. 168–9.

52. Sister Jude, *Freedom to Grow*, pp. 44–6, citing a clinic memorandum from 1945.

53. BCA, BCC/BH 10/1/1/28, Minutes of the Hygiene Sub-Committee of the Education Committee, 9 February 1939; and BCC/BH 10/1/1/29, Minutes of the Hygiene Sub-Committee of the Education Committee, 8 February 1940.

54. Wellcome, SA/SMO/P. 2/22, cutting from the *Jewish Chronicle*, 20 January 1939.

55. CF, series 31, Reports of the General Director, 'Report of the General Director to the Directors of the Commonwealth Fund, April 8th 1937', p. 16; and 'Report of the General Director to the Directors of the Commonwealth Fund, April 20th 1939', pp. 36–7, 31–2.

56. CF, series 7, box 7, folders 51–3, Reports of the Board of Directors, data extracted for relevant years.
57. The Nuffield Foundation, *Report on Grants Made during the Ten Years April 1943 to March 1953* (Oxford: Oxford University Press, 1954), p. 16.
58. Wellcome, GC/186/5, letters 20 January and 1 February 1944, St Loe Strachey to Janet Vaughan.
59. National Association for Mental Health, *First Report: 1946–7* (London: National Association for Mental Health, 1947), pp. 19–20.
60. E. Miller, 'The Future of the Mental Hygiene of Children', in *The Future of Child Guidance in Relation to War Experience*, pp. 18–24, 28–31, on pp. 19, 20, 21, 22, 28.
61. Provisional National Council for Mental Health, *The Sixth Biennial Child Guidance Interclinic Conference* (London: Provisional National Council for Mental Health, 1943), pp. 1–2.
62. Ibid., p. 5.
63. Ibid.
64. Ibid., p. 8.
65. Ibid., p. 14.

6 Child Guidance and the British Welfare State

1. G. Calver, 'Mental Hygiene Reaches the People', *Health Education*, 1:2 (1943), pp. 69–72, on pp. 69, 71, 72.
2. Miss R. Thomas, Child Guidance Council, reported in *Mother and Child*, 14:5 (1943), p. 93.
3. Wellcome, PSY/BPS/1/3/6, Minutes of Meeting of Council, 3 June 1944.
4. TNA, ED 50/274, letter, 2 December 1941, Standing Joint Committee of Working Women's Organisations to the Board of Education.
5. NAS, ED 7/1/49, letter, May 1943, National Union of Women Teachers to Members of Parliament.
6. L. Manning reported in *Mother and Child*, 14:6 (1943), p. 116.
7. LMA, 22.06 LCC, 'Report of the General Sub-Committee of the Education Committee', 14th September and 9th and 23rd November 1943'.
8. NAS, ED 7/1/52, copy of Board of Education document, 'Education after the War', 1941, p. 32.
9. TNA, ED 50/274, Internal Board Memorandum, January 1942, M481/96, 'Schemes for Psychiatric Treatment'.
10. TNA, ED 50/274, letter, 6 October 1942, Board of Education to Ministry of Health.
11. Bodleian Library, University of Oxford, Conservative Party Archives, R. A. Butler Papers (hereafter, Butler Papers), RAB 2/10, 'President's Interview Notes', no. 15, 23 December 1942, p. 1.
12. Norman, *In Way of Understanding*, pp. 138–9, 155.
13. TNA, CAB/66/38/49, Board of Education, 'Educational Reconstruction', paras 93–4.
14. Wellcome, Addis Papers, PP/ADD/H.5, Typescript, 30 September 1944, 'The Work of the Provisional National Council', p. 1.
15. TNA, ED 50/274, letter, 9 May 1942, R. G. Gordon, Child Guidance Council, to President of the Board of Education.
16. TNA, ED 50/274, letter, 13 May 1942, President of the Board of Education to R. G. Gordon.

17. NAS, ED 15/108, 'Scottish Advisory Council on the Treatment and Rehabilitation of Offenders, Notes Submitted by Professor D. K. Henderson, Department of Psychiatry, Edinburgh University: Paper No. 13', [1945]; and 'Minutes of the Twelfth Meeting of the Scottish Advisory Council on the Treatment and Rehabilitation of Offenders, 20 July 1945'. I am grateful to Professor Roger Davison, University of Edinburgh, for alerting me to the work of this committee.

18. This and the following paragraphs derive from TNA, ED 50/274, Board of Education Memorandum, M481/139, 'Child Guidance – General'.

19. Wooldridge, *Measuring the Mind*, pp. 13, 251.

20. D. Thom, 'The 1944 Education Act: The "Art of the Possible"', in H. L. Smith (ed.), *War and Social Change: British Society in the Second World War* (Manchester: Manchester University Press, 1986), pp. 101–28, on p. 109.

21. C. Burt, *The Young Delinquent*, 4th edn (London: University of London Press, 1944), pp. 647–51.

22. 8 & 9 Geo. 6, ch. 37.

23. Parliamentary Debates, 5th series, vol. 410, 1944–5, col. 1269.

24. 7 & 8 Geo 6, ch. 31.

25. TNA, ED 50/274, letter, 26 April 1944, Board of Education to Board of Control.

26. The Ministry of Education, *The Health of the School Child: Report of the Chief Medical Officer of the Ministry of Education for the Years 1939–45*, pp. 68–9.

27. Ministry of Education, *Report of the Committee on Maladjusted Children*, pp. 12–13.

28. Butler Papers, RAB 2/7, 'Memorandum by the President of the Board of Education: Education Bill' to War Cabinet Legislation Committee, 26 November 1943.

29. TNA, ED 50/274, Memorandum, Council of the Royal Medico-Psychological Association, 'Psychiatrists in the Child Guidance Services', [late 1944].

30. MRC, MSS.378/APSW/P/5/3, Minutes of the General Meeting, 20 May 1944, p. 5.

31. Wellcome, SA/SMO/P. 9/22, 'Association of Education Committees: Report of the Child-Guidance Sub-Committee', [1944/5].

32. Wellcome, SA/SMO/P. 9/22, 'Society of Medical Officers of Health: Report of the Child Guidance Sub-Committee of the Association of Education Committees: Comments Submitted by the Child Guidance Sub-Committee of the School Medical Service Group', [1945], pp. 1–2.

33. Wellcome, SA/SMO/P. 9/22, letter, authorship unclear, 11 October 1948.

34. Wellcome, SA/MAC/E.5/6, 'Minutes of a General Meeting of the Association of Psychiatric Social Workers, 31st October 1942', p. 1.

35. 'Report on the National Conference on Maternity and Child Welfare', *Mother and Child*, 15:10 (1945), p. 158.

36. Thomson, *The Problem of Mental Deficiency*, p. 289; Thomson, *Psychological Subjects*, p. 241.

37. BLPES, Central Filing Registry/514/1/G, Sybil Clement Brown, 5 August 1943, 'Notes on Dr Blacker's Memoranda on Regional Psychiatric Services'.

38. Addis, *History of the Child Guidance Movement*, pp. 3, 4; Ministry of Education, *Report of the Committee on Maladjusted Children*, pp. 50–1.

39. Addis, *History of the Child Guidance Movement*, p. 5.

40. C. Webster, 'Psychiatry and the Early National Health Service: The Role of the Mental Health Standing Advisory Committee', in Berrios and Freeman (eds), *150 Years of British Psychiatry*, pp. 103–16, on p. 109.

41. Sampson, *Child Guidance: Its History, Provenance, and Future*, p. 29.

42. W. M. Burbury, 'Introductory', in W. M. Burbury, E. M. Balint and B. J. Yapp, *An Introduction to Child Guidance* (London: Macmillan and Co., 1945), pp. 1–18, on pp. 2, 6, 7.
43. The Ministry of Education, *The Health of the School Child: Report of the Chief Medical Officer for the Ministry of Education for the Years 1939–45*, p. 67.
44. 'International Congress on Mental Health', *BMJ*, 2 (1948), p. 396.
45. Henderson and Gillespie, *A Textbook of Psychiatry for Students and Practitioners*, pp. 629, 11.
46. Ministry of Health, *Report of the Care of Children Committee* (London: HMSO, 1946), pp. 187–91, 68.
47. H. Hendrick, 'Optimism and Hope versus Anxiety and Narcissism: Some Thoughts on Children's Welfare Yesterday and Today', *History of Education*, 36:6 (2007), pp. 747–68, on p. 757.
48. Mayhew, 'Between Love and Aggression', pp. 29–30 and throughout.
49. R. Porter, 'Two Cheers for Psychiatry! The Social History of Mental Disorder in Twentieth Century Britain', in H. Freeman and G. E. Berrios (eds), *150 Years of British Psychiatry Volume II: The Aftermath* (London: Athlone, 1996), pp. 383–406, on p. 308.
50. MRC, MSS.378/APSW/P/5/3, Minutes of the General Meeting, 28 May 1949, p. 3.
51. National Association for Mental Health, *Psychiatric Out-Patient Facilities in the United Kingdom: Part I, Child Guidance Clinics* (London: NAMH, 1950).
52. Ministry of Education, *Report of the Committee on Maladjusted Children*, pp. 13, 98.
53. National Association for Mental Health, *Child Guidance Services in England and Wales, 1955* (London: NAMH, 1955), pp. 38–9, 21–2, 1.
54. Highland Council Archives, Inverness, CI/3/1/65, 'Minutes of the Staffing and Organisation Sub-Committee of the County Council of Inverness', 13 October 1942; and CI/3/1/73, 'Minutes of the Public Health Committee of the County Council of Inverness', 15 October 1946.
55. NAS, ED 28/174, [*c.* 1952], memorandum, 'The Child Guidance Service in Scotland', pp. 1–2.
56. NAS, ED 28/174, 'Notes of a Meeting with Representatives of the Scottish Section of the Council of Professional Psychologists (Mental Health) Held in St. Andrew's House on Monday, 5th March, 1956', p. 2.
57. Thomson, *Psychological Subjects*, p. 202.

7 Child Guidance in Britain at Mid-Century: 'More Akin to Magic than to Medicine'

1. C. Wardle, 'Twentieth Century Influences on the Development in Britain of Services for Child and Adolescent Psychiatry', *British Journal of Psychiatry*, 159 (1991), pp. 53–68, on pp. 58–9.
2. North Wales Mental Hospital Management Committee, *Annual Report for the Year 1954* (Denbigh: North Wales Mental Hospital Management Committee, 1955), pp. 10, 46, 50.
3. Letter, from Edgar McCoy, Dumfries, *BMJ*, 2 (1954), p. 592.
4. Ministry of Health, *Report of the Committee on Social Workers in the Mental Health Services*, p. 12.
5. 'Shortage of Child Psychiatrists in London', *BMJ*, 2 (1951), p. 298.
6. E. M. Creak, 'Refresher Course for General Practitioners: The Nervous Child', *BMJ*, 2 (1951), p. 287.

7. D. Wills, 'Fifty Years of Child Guidance: A Psychologist's View', *Journal of Child Psychotherapy*, 4:4 (1978), pp. 97–102, on pp. 101–2.

8. Wellcome, PSY/BPS/1/3/5, 'Minutes of Meeting of Council, 10 November 1937', 'Minutes of Meeting of Council, 3 October 1942', 'Minutes of Meeting of Council, 28 November 1942' and 'Minutes of Meeting of Council, 3 July 1943'; and PSY/BPS/1/3/6, 'Minutes of Meeting of Council, 8 July 1944'.

9. Hall, 'The Emergence of Clinical Psychology from 1943 to 1958 Part I', pp. 35, 39, 51, 41.

10. National Association for Mental Health, *Ninth Child Guidance Inter-Clinic Conference: Follow-Up on Child Guidance Cases* (London: NAMH, 1951), p. 44.

11. G. Keir, 'Symposium on Psychologists and Psychiatrists in the Child Guidance Service: III – A History of Child Guidance', *British Journal of Educational Psychology*, 22:1 (1952), pp. 5–29, on pp. 26, 5, 11, 13, 26, 28.

12. M. Davidson, 'Symposium on Psychologists and Psychiatrists in the Child Guidance Service: II – The Relation Between Psychologists and Psychiatrists in the Service of Maladjusted Adults and Children', *British Journal of Educational Psychology*, 22:1 (1952), pp. 1–4, on pp. 3, 4.

13. A. Kennedy, 'Symposium on Psychologists and Psychiatrists in the Child Guidance Service: I – Psychologists and Psychiatrists and their General Relationship', *British Journal of Educational Psychology*, 21:3 (1951), pp. 167–71, on pp. 169, 170.

14. R. L. Moody, 'Symposium on Psychologists and Psychiatrists in the Child Guidance Service: V – A Conflict of Disciplines and Personalities', *British Journal of Educational Psychology*, 12:3 (1952), pp. 155–9, on pp. 155, 158, 156.

15. Ibid., pp. 156–9.

16. C. Burt, 'Symposium on Psychologists and Psychiatrists in the Child Guidance Service: VII – Conclusion', *British Journal of Educational Psychology*, 23:1 (1953), pp. 8–28, on pp. 8, 9, 23, 11, 12.

17. Ibid., p. 27.

18. Quoted in Rose, 'Disorders Without Borders?', p. 467.

19. 'Discussion on the Development of Psychiatry within the National Health Service', *Proceedings of the Royal Society of Medicine*, 42 (1949), pp. 365–6.

20. K. Cameron, 'Past and Present Trends in Child Psychiatry', *Journal of Mental Science*, 102 (1956), pp. 599–603, on pp. 600–01.

21. J. Ryle, 'The Meaning of Normal', *Lancet*, 1 (1947), pp. 1–5.

22. Wellcome, SA/SMO/P. 9/22, cutting from *Public Health*, July 1956, p. 193.

23. City and County of Bristol, *The Health of Bristol in 1959*, section F, p. 3.

24. John Rylands Library, University of Manchester, Medical Collection, City of Manchester Education Committee, *Annual Report on the Work of the School Health Service for the Year 1945* (Manchester: City of Manchester Education Committee, 1946), p. 19. It is not clear what, if anything, came of this proposal.

25. Central Library Manchester: Local Studies and Archives, files in series M354/X. A restricted access agreement was signed on 16 August 2006 and the children in the individual files have been anonymized.

26. J. Bowlby, 'The Study and Reduction of Group Tensions in the Family', *Human Relations*, 11:2 (1949), pp. 123–8, on pp. 123, 124–6, 127, 124 – emphasis in the original.

27. Bowlby, 'Introduction to the Papers', in National Association for Mental Health, *11th Inter-Clinic Conference for Staffs of Child Guidance Clinics*, pp. 5–10, on pp. 5, 7.

28. D. Hunter, 'An Approach to Psychotherapeutic Work with Children and Parents', in National Association for Mental Health, *11th Inter-Clinic Conference for Staffs of Child Guidance Clinics*, pp. 11–27, on pp. 12, 14, 11–12.
29. Bowlby, *Child Care and the Growth of Love*, pp. 101–2.
30. D. R. MacCalman, 'Foreword', in A. H. Bowley, *The Natural Development of the Child* (Edinburgh, E. & S. Livingstone, 1947), pp. v–viii, on pp. v, vii.
31. H. Edelston, *The Earliest Stages of Delinquency: A Clinical Study from the Child Guidance Clinic* (Edinburgh: E. & S. Livingstone, 1952), p. 43.
32. K. Cameron, 'Diagnostic Categories in Child Psychiatry', *British Journal of Medical Psychology*, 28:1 (1955), pp. 67–71, on p. 67.
33. 'The Maladjusted Child', *BMJ*, 1 (1956), pp. 217–8.
34. MRC, MSS.378/APSW/P/2/2, APSW, 'Annual Report 1956', p. 6.
35. National Association for Mental Health, *Annual Report, 1956–57* (London: NAMH, 1957), p. 8.
36. National Association for Mental Health, *20th Inter-Clinic Conference for Staffs of Child Guidance Clinics: Evaluation with a View to Action* (London: NAMH, 1956), p. 10.
37. BLPES, R/E97, 'Memorandum Submitted by the National Association for Mental Health to the Committee on Maladjusted Children', 23 June 1952, pp. 5, 3, 6.
38. Wellcome, Addis Papers, PP/ADD/K.2/3, The National Association for Mental Health, *Committee on Maladjusted Children: Memorandum Submitted by the National Association for Mental Health* (London: NAMH, 1952), pp. 1, 2.
39. Wellcome, SA/SMO/P. 9/22, 'Oral Evidence, Given by the Representatives of the Society of Medical Officers of Health, 2nd November, 1951, to the Committee on Maladjusted Children', pp. 4–5.
40. Wellcome, PSY/BPS/1/3/7, 'Minutes of Meeting of Council', 7 July 1951.
41. Wellcome, PSY/BPS/1/3/7, 'Minutes of Meeting of Council', 5 February 1955.
42. Wellcome, Addis Papers, PP/ADD/K.2/3, Royal Medico-Psychological Association, *Memorandum on the 'Report of the Committee on Maladjusted Children': A Memorandum Prepared by the Child Psychiatry Section of the Royal Medico-Psychological Association* (London: Royal Medico-Psychological Association, 1958), p. 1.
43. Ministry of Education, *Report of the Committee on Maladjusted Children*, pp. 1, iv, iii.
44. Wellcome, Addis Papers, PP/ADD/K.2/3, The Magistrates' Association, *Thirty-First Annual Report, 1950–51* (London: The Magistrates' Association, 1951), p. 19.
45. Ministry of Education, *Report of the Committee on Maladjusted Children*, appendix A.
46. Ibid., p. 98.
47. Ibid., pp. 14–15.
48. Ibid., pp. 95, 96, 97, appendix H.
49. Ibid., p. 133.
50. Ibid., pp. 132, 30, 3, appendix F.
51. Ibid., pp. 132, 133, 44, 143.
52. Ibid., pp. 44–5, 50, 43 and ch. 6 and appendix F throughout. Ch. 14 was devoted to the training and supply of child guidance workers.
53. K. McDougall, 'Introduction', in National Association for Mental Health, *Child Guidance – The Changing Scene. Being the Proceedings of the 15th Inter-Clinic Conference* (London: NAMH, 1957), pp. 5–6, on p. 5.
54. Dr E. M. Bartlett, 'A Psychologist Surveys the Changing Scene', in National Association for Mental Health, *Child Guidance – The Changing Scene*, pp. 7–12, on pp. 7, 8, 11, 12.
55. Wooldridge, *Measuring the Mind*, p. 317.

56. Dr G. S. Prince, 'A Psychiatrist Surveys the Changing Scene', in National Association for Mental Health, *Child Guidance – The Changing Scene*, pp. 20–33, on pp. 25, 22 and throughout.

57. Wardle, 'Twentieth Century Influences', p. 59.

58. Prince, 'A Psychiatrist Surveys the Changing Scene', pp. 25, 32.

59. H. Freeman, 'Psychiatry and the State in Britain', (ed) M. Gijswijt-Hofstra, H. Oosterhuis, J. Vijselaar and H. Freeman (eds), *Psychiatric Cultures Compared: Psychiatry and Mental Health Care in the Twentieth Century* (Amsterdam: Amsterdam University Press, 2005), pp. 116–40, on pp. 126–32; V. Long, *Destigmatising Mental Illness? Professional Politics and Public Education in Britain, 1870–1970* (Manchester: Manchester University Press, forthcoming), ch. 3. I am grateful to Dr Long for letting me see a pre-publication draft of this volume.

60. M. R. Barnes, 'A Psychiatric Social Worker Surveys the Changing Scene', in National Association for Mental Health, *Child Guidance – The Changing Scene*, pp. 13–19, on pp. 14–15.

61. Ibid., pp. 16, 17.

62. R. S. Addis, 'Social Work in the Mental Health Field in the United Kingdom', *Journal of Psychiatric Social Work*, 22:2 (1953), pp. 82–90, on p. 85.

Conclusion: 'The Dangerous Age of Childhood'

1. Wellcome, Addis Papers, PP/ADD/K.2/3, Royal Medico-Psychological Association, *Memorandum on the 'Report of the Committee on Maladjusted Children: A Memorandum Prepared by the Child Psychiatry Section of the Royal Medico-Psychological Association'*, pp. 4, 5–6.

2. BLPES, R/D499, National Association for Mental Health, *Child Guidance and Child Psychiatry as an Integral Part of Community Services* (London: NAMH, 1965), pp. 4, 7.

3. I am grateful to Professor John Hall for this point.

4. Rosenberg, 'Contested Boundaries', pp. 418–9.

5. See J. Welshman, *Underclass: A History of the Excluded, 1880–2000* (London: Hambledon Continuum, 2006), ch. 4.

6. See, for instance, the PSW Bridget Yapp's description of her duties: B. J. Yapp, 'Methods of Examination (1). Work of the Psychiatric Social Worker', in Burbury, Balint and Yapp (eds), *An Introduction to Child Guidance*, pp. 99–110.

7. J. Welshman, 'Rhetoric and Reality: Community Care in England and Wales, 1948', in P. Bartlett and D. Wright (eds), *Outside the Walls of the Asylum: The History of Care in the Community, 1750–2000* (London: Athlone, 1999), pp. 204–26, on p. 210.

8. I am grateful to Sister Gail Taylor, Notre Dame Centre, Glasgow for this point.

9. Rose, 'Disorders Without Borders?', p. 479.

10. I am grateful to a correspondent, herself a former clinic attendee and to colleagues in the Social Work Department, Glasgow Caledonian University for the point about school stigma.

11. Plant, *Mom*, p. 10 and throughout; Jones, '"Mother Made Me Do It"', p. 101 and throughout.

12. See, for social work in a complementary field, P. Starkey, 'The Feckless Mother: Women, Poverty and Social Workers in Wartime and Post-War England', *Women's History Review*, 9:3 (2000), pp. 539–57.

13. B. Wootton, *Social Science and Social Pathology* (London: George Allen and Unwin, 1959), pp. 270–1, 331, 337–9, 330.
14. J. Stewart, '"The Dangerous Age of Childhood": Child Guidance in Britain *c.* 1918–1955', www.historyandpolicy.org/papers [posted October 2012].

Appendix 2: Cameron's Classification System, 1955

1. This is a condensed version of K. Cameron, 'Diagnostic Categories in Child Psychiatry', *British Journal of Medical Psychology*, 28:1 (1955), pp. 67–71.
2. Cameron notes that the term 'emotional maturity' is difficult and 'emphasizes our lack of standards of emotional development'. However, it still needs to be addressed, and one mechanism is the 'standards of the observer'.

WORKS CITED

Primary Sources

Archives and Special Collections

Birmingham City Archives, BCC/BH

The British Library of Political and Economic Science, Central Filing Registry/514/1

The British Library of Political and Economic Science, Minutes of School Committees/16

The British Library of Political and Economic Science, HQ/60

The British Library of Political and Economic Science, R/D499

The British Library of Political and Economic Science, R/E97

Central Library Manchester: Local Studies and Archives, Series M354/X

Conservative Party Archives, R. A. Butler Papers, Bodleian Library, University of Oxford, RAB 2/7, RAB 2/10

Dundee City Archives, Minutes of a Meeting of the Education Committee

Dundee City Archives, TC/SF/Ed53

Dundee University Archives, RU565/1

Edinburgh City Archives, Council Records

Edinburgh City Archives, SL 164/1/8

Glasgow University Archives and Business Records Centre, DC 130/1/1

Glasgow University Archives and Business Records Centre, UGC 58/1/2/1

Highland Council Archives, Inverness, CI/3/1/65 and 73

John Rylands Library, University of Manchester, Archives and Special Collections

John Rylands Library, University of Manchester, Medical Collection

Labour Party Archives, People's History Museum, Manchester

Liverpool Local Record Office, 352 MIN/EDU

Liverpool Local Record Office, HQ360.5 QUA

London Metropolitan Archives, 22.06 LCC

London Metropolitan Archives, E/NOR/Y/12

London Metropolitan Archives, LCC EO/WEL/1/61

The Mitchell Library, City Archives, Glasgow, D-TC 7/7/13

Modern Records Centre, University of Warwick, MSS.378/APSW/P

The National Archives, London, CAB/66/38/49

The National Archives, London, ED 50/48, ED 50/102, ED 50/273, ED 50/274

The National Archives, London, MH 57/291

The National Archives of Scotland, ED 7/1/49, ED 7/1/52

The National Archives of Scotland, ED 15/108

The National Archives of Scotland, ED 28/174

The National Library of Scotland, Acc.7170

Oxfordshire Local Studies Centre, Oxford, P OXFO/371.26

The Rockefeller Archive Center, New York, Commonwealth Fund Archives, Series 2, 7, 16, 31

Scottish Catholic Archives, Edinburgh, DE 122, DE 125

University of Liverpool Archives and Special Collections, EX 65

University of Liverpool Archives and Special Collections, D.191/20/1

Wellcome Library, London, Addis Papers, PP/ADD

Wellcome Library, London, Bowlby Papers, PP/BOW

Wellcome Library, London, GC/186/5

Wellcome Library, London, MS.7913

Wellcome Library, London, PSY/BPS

Wellcome Library, London, SA/SMO

Periodicals

Archives of Diseases in Childhood, 1935

British Journal of Educational Psychology, 1931, 1933, 1942, 1951, 1952, 1953

British Journal of Medical Psychology, 1929, 1955

British Medical Journal, 1929, 1930, 1931, 1932, 1933, 1948, 1951, 1954, 1956

Child Life, 1925, 1933, 1937, 1938

Child Life Quarterly, 1933

Edinburgh Medical Journal, 1931

Glasgow Medical Journal, 1923

Glasgow Observer, 1931

Health Education, 1943

Human Relations, 1949

International Journal of Psychoanalysis, 1940

Journal of Child Psychotherapy, 1978

Journal of Mental Science, 1939, 1956

Journal of Psychiatric Social Work, 1953

Journal of the Royal Institute of Public Health and Hygiene, 1937

Lancet, 1947

Liverpool Quarterly, 1933

Mental Welfare, 1929, 1935, 1936, 1937, 1938

Mother and Child, 1930, 1931, 1932, 1933, 1934, 1937, 1938, 1939, 1942, 1943, 1944, 1945, 1955

National Froebel Foundation Bulletin, 1941

Proceedings of the Royal Society of Medicine, 1930, 1931, 1949, 1958

Smith College Studies in Social Work, 1930

Tablet, 1930, 1938

Annual Reports

Board of Education, 1927, 1934

Child Guidance Council, 1933, 1934, 1935, 1936, 1938, 1939

City of Manchester Education Committee, 1939, 1940, 1941, 1945

Commonwealth Fund, 1929, 1934, 1938, 1943, 1944

Edinburgh Catholic Child Guidance Clinic, 1934–5

Liverpool Child Guidance Council, 1933

London Child Guidance Clinic, 1929–31

The Magistrates' Association, 1950–1

Ministry of Education, 1939–1945

National Association for Mental Health, 1946–7, 1956–7

North Wales Mental Hospital Management Committee, 1954

Notre Dame Child Guidance Clinic, 1933–4, 1938–9

Provisional National Council for Mental Health, 1943

Printed Sources

Addis, R. S., *History of the Child Guidance Movement* (London: NAMH, 1952).

Ashdown, M. and S. C. Brown, *Social Service and Mental Health: An Essay on Psychiatric Social Workers* (London: Routledge and Kegan Paul, 1953).

Barnes, M. R., 'A Psychiatric Social Worker Surveys the Changing Scene', in National Association for Mental Health, *Child Guidance – The Changing Scene. Being the Proceedings of the 15th Inter-Clinic Conference* (London: NAMH, 1957), pp. 13–19.

Bartlett, Dr E. M., 'A Psychologist Surveys the Changing Scene', in National Association for Mental Health, *Child Guidance – The Changing Scene*, pp. 7–12.

Bodman, F., 'Enemy Action', in *The Future of Child Guidance in Relation to War Experience* (London: The Child Guidance Council, 1941), pp. 1–7.

Bowlby, J., 'Psychological Aspects', in R. Padley and M. Cole (eds), *Evacuation Survey* (London: George Routledge and Sons, 1940), pp. 186–96.

—, *Child Care and the Growth of Love* (Harmondsworth: Penguin Books, 1953).

—, 'Introduction to the Papers', in National Association for Mental Health, *11th Inter-Clinic Conference for Staffs of Child Guidance Clinics: The Family Approach to Child Guidance – Therapeutic Techniques* (London: NAMH, 1955), pp. 5–10.

Boyd, W., 'Preventive Work with Problem Children', in W. Boyd (ed.), *Towards a New Education* (London: Knopf, 1930), pp. 289–90.

Brown, S. C., 'The Methods of Social Case Workers', in F. C. Bartlett, M. Ginsberg, E. J. Lindgren, R. H. Thouless and E. C. Cull (eds), *The Study of Society: Methods and Problems* (London: Kegan Paul, Trench, Trubner and Co., 1939), pp. 379–401.

Burbury, W. M., 'Introductory', in W. M. Burbury, E. M. Balint and B. J. Yapp, *An Introduction to Child Guidance* (London: Macmillan and Co., 1945), pp. 1–18.

—, E. M. Balint and B. J. Yapp, *An Introduction to Child Guidance* (London: Macmillan and Co., 1945).

Burt, C., *The Young Delinquent*, 4th edn (London: University of London Press, 1944).

— (ed.), *How the Mind Works*, 2nd edn (London: George Allen and Unwin, 1945, 1st edn 1933).

Cameron, A. C., 'Education in the City of Oxford', in A. C. Cameron (ed.), *Oxford 1935: A Souvenir of the World Educational Conferences* (Oxford: Oxford University Press, 1935), pp. 245–54.

Child Guidance Council, *List of Recommended Books on Child Psychology, with Annotations* (London: Child Guidance Council, 1935).

—, *Report of the Inter-Clinic Conference 1935* (London: The Child Guidance Council, 1935).

—, *Proceedings of the Child Guidance Inter-Clinic Conference of Great Britain 1939* (London: The Child Guidance Council, 1939), pp. 98–9.

City and Council of Bristol, *The Health of Bristol in 1959* (Bristol: City and County of Bristol, 1960).

City of Dundee, *Report of the Medical Officer of Health for the Year Ending 31st December, 1936* (Dundee: Dundee City Council, 1937).

Collins, M. and J. Drever, *Psychology and Practical Life* (London: University of London Press, 1936).

The Commonwealth Fund, *Historical Sketch, 1918–1962* (New York: The Commonwealth Fund, 1963).

Cook, P. H., *The Theory and Technique of Child Guidance* (Melbourne: Australian Council for Educational Research/Melbourne University Press, 1944).

Crowley, Dr R. H., *Child Guidance Clinics, with Special Reference to American Experience* (London: Child Guidance Council, 1928).

Dickson, M. D. L., *Child Guidance* (London: Sands and Co., 1938).

Drever, J. and M. Drummond, *The Psychology of the Pre-School Child* (London: Partridge, 1929).

Durbin, E. F. M. and J. Bowlby, *Personal Aggressiveness and War* (London: Kegan Paul, Trench, Trubner and Co., 1939), pp. 98–9.

Edelston, H., *The Earliest Stages of Delinquency: A Clinical Study from the Child Guidance Clinic* (Edinburgh: E. & S. Livingstone, 1952).

The Feversham Committee, *The Voluntary Mental Health Services* (London: The Feversham Committee, 1939).

French, L. M., *Psychiatric Social Work* (New York: The Commonwealth Fund, 1940).

Freud, A., 'The Theory of Children's Analysis', in A. Freud, *The Psycho-Analytical Treatment of Children: Technical Lectures and Essays* (London: Imago, 1946), pp. 55–64.

— and D. Burlingham, *Infants without Families and Reports of the Hampstead Nurseries, 1939–1945* (London: The Hogarth Press, 1974).

Glasgow University Settlement, *Social Services for Children and Young People: Glasgow 1936–37* (Glasgow: Glasgow University Settlement, 1937).

Gordon, R. G., 'Foreword', in R. G. Gordon (ed.), *A Survey of Child Psychiatry* (London: Oxford University Press, 1939), pp. v–viii.

Henderson, D. K. and R. D. Gillespie, *A Textbook of Psychiatry for Students and Practitioners*, 7th edn (London: Oxford University Press, 1950).

Hunter, D., 'An Approach to Psychotherapeutic Work with Children and Parents', in National Association for Mental Health, *11th Inter-Clinic Conference for Staffs of Child Guidance Clinics: The Family Approach to Child Guidance – Therapeutic Techniques*, pp. 11–27.

Isaacs, S. (ed.), *The Cambridge Evacuation Survey: A Wartime Study in Social Welfare and Education* (London: Methuen, 1941).

Jewish Health Organisation of Great Britain, *The East London Child Guidance Clinic: Honorary Director's Report, 1927–1932* (London: Jewish Health Organisation of Great Britain, 1933).

Jones, J. T., *History of the Corporation of Birmingham, Vol. V, Part I* (Birmingham: General Purposes Committee Birmingham Corporation, 1940).

Kenna, J. C., *Educational and Psychological Problems of Evacuation: An Analysis of Experience in England* (Melbourne: Australian Council for Educational Research, 1942).

Klein, M., *The Psychoanalysis of Children* (London: The Hogarth Press, 1932).

The Labour Party, *A Children's Charter* (London: The Labour Party, 1937).

London Children in War-Time Oxford: A Survey of Social and Educational Results of Evacuation (London: Oxford University Press, 1947).

Macadam, E., *The New Philanthropy: A Study in the Relations between the Statutory and Voluntary Social Services* (London: George Allen and Unwin, 1934).

McCallum, C., 'Nerston Residential Clinic: An Experiment in Child Guidance', in W. Boyd (ed.), *Evacuation in Scotland: A Record of Events and Experiments* (Bickley: University of London Press, 1944), pp. 170–91.

MacCalman, D. R., 'The General Management of Maladjustment in Children', in R. G. Gordon (ed.), *A Survey of Child Psychiatry* (London: Oxford University Press, 1939), pp. 257–68.

—, 'Foreword', in A. H. Bowley, *The Natural Development of the Child* (Edinburgh, E. & S. Livingstone, 1947), pp. v–viii.

McDougall, K., 'Introduction', in National Association for Mental Health, *Child Guidance – The Changing Scene*, pp. 5–6.

Macgregor, Sir A., *Public Health in Glasgow, 1905–1946* (Edinburgh: E. & S. Livingstone, 1967).

Meyer, A., *The Collected Papers of Adolf Meyer: Volume 4, Mental Hygiene*, ed. E. Winters (Baltimore, MD: Johns Hopkins Press, 1952).

Miller, E., 'The Future of the Mental Hygiene of Children', in *The Future of Child Guidance in Relation to War Experience* (London: The Child Guidance Council, 1941), pp. 18–24, 28–31.

Ministry of Education, *Report of the Committee on Maladjusted Children* (London: HMSO, 1955).

Ministry of Health, *Report of the Care of Children Committee* (London: HMSO, 1946).

—, *Report of the Committee on Social Workers in the Mental Health Services* (London: HMSO, 1951).

Moodie, W. *Child Guidance by Team Work* (London: Child Guidance Council, 1931).

—, *The London Child Guidance Clinic: A Survey* (London; London Child Guidance Clinic, [1935/6]).

—, *The Doctor and the Difficult Child*, 2nd edn (New York: The Commonwealth Fund, 1947).

National Association for Mental Health, *Psychiatric Out-Patient Facilities in the United Kingdom: Part 1, Child Guidance Clinics* (London: NAMH, 1950).

—, *Ninth Child Guidance Inter-Clinic Conference: Follow-Up on Child Guidance Cases* (London: NAMH, 1951), p. 44.

—, *11th Inter-Clinic Conference for Staffs of Child Guidance Clinics: The Family Approach to Child Guidance – Therapeutic Techniques* (London: NAMH, 1955).

—, *Child Guidance Services in England and Wales, 1955* (London: NAMH, 1955).

—, *20th Inter-Clinic Conference for Staffs of Child Guidance Clinics: Evaluation with a View to Action* (London: NAMH, 1956).

—, *Child Guidance – The Changing Scene. Being the Proceedings of the 15th Inter-Clinic Conference* (London: NAMH, 1957).

—, *Child Guidance and Child Psychiatry as an Integral Part of Community Services* (London: NAMH, 1965).

The Nuffield Foundation, *Report on Grants Made during the Ten Years April 1943 to March 1953* (Oxford: Oxford University Press, 1954).

Pinsent, E. F., *The Mental Health Services in Oxford City, Oxfordshire and Berkshire* (Oxford: Oxford University Press, 1937).

Prince, Dr G. S., 'A Psychiatrist Surveys the Changing Scene', in National Association for Mental Health, *Child Guidance – The Changing Scene. Being the Proceedings of the 15th Inter-Clinic Conference*, pp. 20–33.

Proceedings of the National Conference of Social Work (Chicago, IL: University of Chicago Press, 1931).

Provisional National Council for Mental Health, *The Sixth Biennial Child Guidance Inter-clinic Conference* (London: Provisional National Council for Mental Health, 1943).

Report of the Institution and Development of the Child Guidance Clinic at Guy's Hospital London, 1930–1936 (London: Guy's Hospital, [1936/7]).

Rickman, J., 'Preface', in J. Rickman (ed.), *On the Bringing Up of Children* (London: Paul, Trench and Trubner, 1936), pp. 7–14.

St Loe Strachey, Mrs, *Borrowed Children: A Popular Account of Some Evacuation Problems and their Remedies* (New York: The Commonwealth Fund, 1940).

Scottish Education Department, *Report of the Committee of Council on Education in Scotland for the Year 1938* (Edinburgh: HMSO, 1939).

Shapiro, P. C., *How Child Guidance Contributes to Mental Health* (London: Child Guidance Council, 1933).

Sister Marie Hilda, *Child Guidance* (London: Catholic Truth Society, 1950).

Swift, S. H., *Training in Psychiatric Social Work at the Institute for Child Guidance, 1927–1933* (New York: The Commonwealth Fund, 1934).

Titmuss, R., *Problems of Social Policy* (London: HMSO, 1950), pp. 102–3.

Valentine, C. W., *The Difficult Child and the Problem of Discipline* (London: Methuen, 1940).

Witmer, H. L., *Psychiatric Clinics for Children: With Special Reference to State Programs* (New York: The Commonwealth Fund, 1940).

Yapp, B. J., 'Methods of Examination (1). Work of the Psychiatric Social Worker', in Burbury, Balint and Yapp (eds), *An Introduction to Child Guidance*, pp. 99–110.

Secondary Sources

Angel, K., 'Defining Psychiatry: Aubrey Lewis's 1938 Report and the Rockefeller Foundation', in K. Angel, E. Jones and M. Neve (eds), *European Psychiatry on the Eve of War: Aubrey Lewis, the Maudsley Hospital and the Rockefeller Foundation in the 1930s, Medical History Supplement 22* (2003), pp. 39–56.

Armstrong, D., 'The Rise of Surveillance Medicine', *Sociology of Health and Illness*, 17:3 (1995), pp. 393–404.

—, *A New History of Identity: A Sociology of Medical Knowledge* (Basingstoke: Palgrave, 2002).

Bakker, N., 'Health and the Medicalisation of Advice to Parents in the Netherlands, 1890–1950', in M. Gijswijt-Hofstra and H. Marland (eds), *Cultures of Child Health in Britain and the Netherlands in the Twentieth Century* (Amsterdam: Rodopi, 2003), pp. 127–48.

—, 'Child Guidance and Mental Health in the Netherlands', *Paedagogica Historica*, 42:6 (2006), pp. 769–91.

Bowlby, J., 'A Historical Perspective on Child Guidance', *Child Guidance Trust: Newsletter No. 3* (June 1987), pp. 1–2.

Bowler, P. J., 'Experts and Publishers: Writing Popular Science in Early Twentieth-Century Britain, Writing Popular History of Science Now', *British Journal for the History of Science*, 39:2 (2006), pp. 159–87.

Burnham, D., 'Selective Memory: A Note on Social Work Historiography', *British Journal of Social Work*, 41:1 (2011), pp. 5–21.

Cohen, S., 'The Mental Hygiene Movement, the Development of Personality and the School: The Medicalization of American Education', *History of Education Quarterly*, 23:2 (1983), pp. 123–49.

Cook, H., *The Long Sexual Revolution: English Women, Sex, and Contraception, 1800–1975* (Oxford: Oxford University Press, 2004), pp. 147, 210.

Cooter, R., 'In the Name of the Child Beyond', in M. Gijswit-Hofstra and H. Marland (eds), *Cultures of Child Health in Britain and the Netherlands in the Twentieth Century*, pp. 287–96.

Dell, G., 'Thirty Years of Child Guidance: The Development of the Glasgow Child Guidance Service', *Scottish Educational Research*, 1:3 (1969), pp. 32–8.

Dicks, H. V., *Fifty Years of the Tavistock Clinic* (London: Routledge and Kegan Paul, 1970).

Evans, B., et al., 'Managing the "Unmanageable": Interwar Child Psychiatry at the Maudsley Hospital, London', *History of Psychiatry*, 19:4 (2008), pp. 454–75.

Freeman, H., 'Psychiatry and the State in Britain', in M. Gijswijt-Hofstra, H. Oosterhuis, J. Vijselaar and H. Freeman (eds), *Psychiatric Cultures Compared: Psychiatry and Mental Health Care in the Twentieth Century* (Amsterdam: Amsterdam University Press, 2005), pp. 116–40.

Friedman, L. J. and M. D. McGarvie (eds), *Charity, Philanthropy, and Civility in American History* (Cambridge: Cambridge University Press, 2003).

Gelder, M., 'Adolf Meyer and his Influence on British Psychiatry', in G. E. Berrios and H. Freeman (eds), *150 Years of British Psychiatry* (London: Athlone, 1991), pp. 419–35.

Gijswijt-Hofstra, M. and H. Marland (eds), *Cultures of Child Health in Britain and the Netherlands in the Twentieth Century* (Amsterdam: Rodopi, 2003).

Graebner, W., 'The Unstable World of Benjamin Spock: Social Engineering in a Democratic Culture, 1917–1950', *Journal of American History*, 67: 3 (1980), pp. 612–29.

Grob, G. N., *The Mad Among Us: A History of the Care of America's Mentally Ill* (New York: The Free Press, 1994).

Grosvenor, I. and K. Myers, 'Progressivism, Control and Correction: Local Education Authorities and Educational Policy in Twentieth Century England', *Paedagogica Historica*, 42:1, 42:2 (2006), pp. 225–47.

Hall, J., 'The Emergence of Clinical Psychology in Britain from 1943 to 1958 Part 1: Core Tasks and the Professsionalisation Process', *History and Philosophy of Psychology*, 9:1 (2007), pp. 29–55.

Hammack, D. C., 'Failure and Resilience: Pushing the Limits in Depression and Wartime', in L. J. Friedman and M. D. McGarvie (eds), *Charity, Philanthropy, and Civility in American History* (Cambridge: Cambridge University Press, 2003), pp. 263–80.

Harvey, A. McG. and S. L. Abrams, *'For the Welfare of Mankind': The Commonwealth Fund and American Medicine* (Baltimore, MD: Johns Hopkins University Press, 1986).

Hayes, S., 'Rabbits and Rebels: The Medicalisation of Maladjusted Children in Mid-Twentieth Century Britain', in M. Jackson (ed.), *Health and the Modern Home* (London: Routledge, 2007), pp. 128–52.

Hendrick, H., *Child Welfare: Historical Dimensions, Contemporary Debate* (Bristol: The Policy Press, 2003).

—, 'Optimism and Hope versus Anxiety and Narcissism: Some Thoughts on Children's Welfare Yesterday and Today', *History of Education*, 36:6 (2007), pp. 747–68.

Horn, M., 'Inventing the Problem Child: "At Risk" Children in the Child Guidance Movement of the 1920s and 1930s', in R. Wollons (ed.), *Children at Risk in America: History, Concepts, and Public Policy* (Albany: State University of New York Press, 1993), pp. 141–56.

Hurl, C., 'Urine Trouble: A Social History of Bedwetting and its Regulation', *History of the Human Sciences*, 24:2 (2011), pp. 48–64.

Jones, E. H., *Margery Fry: The Essential Amateur* (York: The Ebor Press, 1966).

Jones, K., 'Law and Mental Health', in G. Berrios and H. Freeman (eds), *150 Years of British Psychiatry* (London: Gaskell, 1991), pp. 89–102.

Jones, K. W., '"Mother Made Me Do It": Mother-Blaming and the Women of Child Guidance', in M. Ladd-Taylor and L. Umansky (eds), *'Bad' Mothers: The Politics of Blame in Twentieth-Century America* (New York: New York University Press, 1998), pp. 99–124.

—, *Taming the Troublesome Child: American Families, Child Guidance, and the Limits of Psychiatric Authority* (Cambridge, MA: Harvard University Press, 1999).

Jones, M., *Holding On* (London: Quartet Books, 1973).

Jordanova, L., 'The Social Construction of Medical Knowledge', *Social History of Medicine*, 8:3 (2005), pp. 361–81.

Kuklick, H., *The Savage Within: The Social History of British Anthropology, 1885–1945* (Cambridge: Cambridge University Press, 1991).

Lane, C., *Shyness: How Normal Behaviour Became a Sickness* (New Haven, CT: Yale University Press, 2007).

Lawrence, C., *Rockefeller Money, the Laboratory, and Medicine in Edinburgh, 1919–1930: New Science in an Old Country* (Rochester, NY: University of Rochester Press, 2005).

Long, V., '"Often There is a Good Deal to be Done, But Socially Rather than Medically": The Psychiatric Social Worker as Social Therapist, 1945–1970', *Medical History*, 55:2 (2011), pp. 223–39.

—, *Destigmatising Mental Illness? Professional Politics and Public Education in Britain, 1870–1970* (Manchester: Manchester University Press, forthcoming).

Lubove, R., *The Professional Altruist: The Emergence of Social Work as a Career, 1880–1930* (Cambridge, MA: Harvard University Press, 1965).

Ludvigsen, K. and Å. A. Seip, 'The Establishing of Norwegian Child Psychiatry: Ideas, Pioneers, and Institutions', *History of Psychiatry*, 20:1 (2009), pp. 5–26.

Lunbeck, E., *The Psychiatric Persuasion: Knowledge, Gender and Power in Modern America* (Princeton, NJ: Princeton University Press, 1994).

McCallum, Sister J., et al., 'Foundations', in *The Notre Dame Centre, Freedom to Grow: Celebrating 75 Years of the Notre Dame Centre in Glasgow* (Glasgow: The Publishing Cupboard, 2007), pp. 8–21.

Mayhew, B., 'Between Love and Aggression: The Politics of John Bowlby', *History of the Human Sciences*, 19:4 (2006), pp. 19–35.

Norman, P., *In Way of Understanding: Part of a Life – Lantern Slides in a Rough Time Sequence* (Godalming: The Foxbury Press, 1982).

Nottingham, C., 'The Rise of the Insecure Professionals', *International Review of Social History*, 52:3 (2007), pp. 445–75.

Nuttall, J., '"Psychological Socialist"; "Militant Moderate": Evan Durbin and the Politics of Synthesis', *Labour History Review*, 68:2 (2003), pp. 235–52.

Obituary, 'Tilda Goldberg', *Guardian*, 10 January 2005, p. 19.

Overy, R., *The Morbid Age: Britain between the Wars* (London: Allen Lane, 2009).

Paterson, L., *Scottish Education in the Twentieth Century* (Edinburgh: Edinburgh University Press, 2003), pp. 47–8.

Plant, R. J., *Mom: The Transformation of Motherhood in Modern America* (Chicago, IL: University of Chicago Press, 2010).

Porter, R., 'Two Cheers for Psychiatry! The Social History of Mental Disorder in Twentieth Century Britain', in H. Freeman and G. E. Berrios (eds), *150 Years of British Psychiatry Volume II: The Aftermath* (London: Athlone, 1996), pp. 383–406.

Richards, G., 'Britain on the Couch: The Popularization of Psychoanalysis in Britain, 1918–1940', *Science in Context*, 13:2 (2000), pp. 183–230.

Rodgers, D. T., *Atlantic Crossings: Social Politics in a Progressive Age* (Cambridge, MA: Harvard University Press, 1998).

Rose, N., *The Psychological Complex: Psychology, Politics and Society in England, 1869–1939* (London: Routledge and Kegan Paul, 1985).

—, *Governing the Soul: The Shaping of the Private Self* (London: Routledge, 1989).

—, 'Engineering the Human Soul: Analyzing Psychological Expertise', *Science in Context*, 5:2 (1992), pp. 351–69.

—, 'Disorders Without Borders? The Expanding Scope of Psychiatric Practice', *BioSocieties*, 1:4 (2006), pp. 465–84.

Rosenberg, C. E., 'Holism in Twentieth Century Medicine', in C. Lawrence and G. Weisz (eds), *Greater Than the Parts: Holism in Biomedicine, 1920–1950* (New York: Oxford University Press, 1998), pp. 335–55.

—, 'Pathologies of Progress: The Idea of Civilization as Risk', *Bulletin of the History of Medicine*, 72:4 (1998), pp. 714–30.

—, 'What is Disease? In Memory of Owsei Temkin', *Bulletin of the History of Medicine*, 77:3 (2003), pp. 491–505.

—, 'Contested Boundaries: Psychiatry, Disease and Diagnosis', *Perspectives in Biology and Medicine*, 49:3 (2006), pp. 407–24.

Rosenberg, E. S., 'Missions to the World: American Philanthropy Abroad', in Friedman and McGarvie (eds), *Charity, Philanthropy, and Civility in American History*, pp. 241–58.

Sampson, O., *Child Guidance: Its History, Provenance and Future* (London: British Psychological Society, 1980).

Shorter, E., *A History of Psychiatry: From the Era of the Asylum to the Age of Prozac* (New York: John Wiley and Sons, 1997).

Sister Jude, *Freedom to Grow: Sister Marie Hilda's Vision of Child Guidance* (Glasgow: John S. Burns and Sons, 1981).

Starkey, P., 'The Feckless Mother: Women, Poverty and Social Workers in Wartime and Post-War England', *Women's History Review*, 9:3 (2000), pp. 539–57.

Stearns, P., 'Defining Happy Childhoods: Assessing a Recent Change', *Journal of the History of Childhood and Youth*, 3:2 (2010), pp. 165–86.

Stewart, J., '"An Enigma to their Parents": The Founding and Aims of the Notre Dame Child Guidance Clinic, Glasgow', *Innes Review*, 57:1 (2006), pp. 54–76.

—, 'Child Guidance in Interwar Scotland: International Context and Domestic Concerns', *Bulletin of the History of Medicine*, 80:3 (2006), pp. 513–39.

—, '"I Thought You Would Want to Come and See his Home ...": Child Guidance and Psychiatric Social Work in Inter-War Britain', in M. Jackson (ed.), *Health and the Modern Home* (London: Routledge, 2007), pp. 111–27.

—, 'The Scientific Claims of British Child Guidance, 1918–45', *British Journal for the History of Science*, 42:3 (2009), pp. 407–32.

—, 'Child Guidance in Scotland 1918–55: Psychiatry versus Psychology?', *History and Philosophy of Psychology*, 12:2 (2010), pp. 26–36.

—, '"The Dangerous Age of Childhood": Child Guidance and the "Normal" Child in Great Britain, 1920–1950', *Paedagogica Historica*, 47:6 (2011), pp. 785–803.

—, '"The Dangerous Age of Childhood": Child Guidance in Britain *c.* 1918–1955', www.historyandpolicy.org/papers [posted October 2012].

Sturdy, S. and R. Cooter, 'Science, Scientific Management, and the Transformation of Medicine in Britain, *c.* 1870–1950', *History of Science*, 36:4 (1998), pp. 421–66.

Thom, D., 'The 1944 Education Act: The "Art of the Possible"', in H. L. Smith (ed.), *War and Social Change: British Society in the Second World War* (Manchester: Manchester University Press, 1986), pp. 101–28.

—, 'Wishes, Anxiety, Play, and Gestures: Child Guidance in Inter-War England', in R. Cooter (ed.), *In the Name of the Child: Health and Welfare, 1880–1940* (London: Routledge, 1992), pp. 200–19.

Thomson, M., 'Mental Hygiene as an International Movement', in P. Weindling (ed.), *International Health Organisations and Movements* (Cambridge: Cambridge University Press, 1995), pp. 283–304.

—, *The Problem of Mental Deficiency: Eugenics, Democracy, and Social Policy in Britain, 1870–1959* (Oxford: Oxford University Press, 1998), pp. 165–6.

—'Psychology and the "Consciousness of Modernity" in Early Twentieth Century Britain', in M. Daunton and B. Rieger (eds), *Meanings of Modernity: Britain from the Late-Victorian Era to World War II* (Oxford: Berg, 2001), pp. 97–144.

—, *Psychological Subjects: Identity, Culture, and Health in Twentieth Century Britain* (Oxford: Oxford University Press, 2006).

Timms, N., *Psychiatric Social Work in Great Britain, 1939–1962* (London: Routledge and Kegan Paul, 1964).

Turmel, A., *A Historical Sociology of Childhood* (Cambridge: Cambridge University Press, 2008).

Urwin, C., 'Margaret Lowenfeld', in C. Urwin and J. Hood-Williams (eds), *Selected Papers of Margaret Lowenfeld* (London: Free Association Books, 1988), part 1, pp. 3–139.

— and E. Sharland, 'From Bodies to Minds in Childcare Literature: Advice to Parents in Inter-War Britain', in R. Cooter (ed.), *In the Name of the Child: Health and Welfare, 1880–1940* (London: Routledge, 1992), pp. 174–99.

van Dijken, S., R. van der Veer, M. van Ijzendoorn and H.-J. Kuipers, 'Bowlby before Bowlby: The Sources of an Intellectual Departure in Psychoanalysis and Psychology', *Journal of the History of the Behavioural Sciences*, 34:3 (1998), pp. 247–69.

Wardle, C., 'Twentieth Century Influences on the Development in Britain of Services for Child and Adolescent Psychiatry', *British Journal of Psychiatry*, 159 (1991), pp. 53–68.

Webster, C., 'Psychiatry and the Early National Health Service: The Role of the Mental Health Standing Advisory Committee', in G. E. Berrios and H. Freeman (eds), *150 Years of British Psychiatry* (London: Gaskell, 1991), pp. 103–16.

Welshman, J., 'Rhetoric and Reality: Community Care in England and Wales, 1948', in P. Bartlett and D. Wright (eds), *Outside the Walls of the Asylum: The History of Care in the Community, 1750–2000* (London: Athlone, 1999), pp. 204–26.

—, *Underclass: A History of the Excluded, 1880–2000* (London: Hambledon Continuum, 2006).

—, *Churchill's Children: The Evacuee Experience in Wartime Britain* (Oxford: Oxford University Press, 2010).

Wheatcroft, S., 'Cured by Kindness? Child Guidance Services during the Second World War', in A. Borsay and P. Dale (eds), *Disabled Children: Contested Caring, 1850–1979* (London: Pickering & Chatto, 2012), pp. 145–57.

Wooldridge, A., *Measuring the Mind: Education and Psychology in England, c. 1860–c. 1990* (Cambridge: Cambridge University Press, 1994).

Wootton, B., *Social Science and Social Pathology* (London: George Allen and Unwin, 1959).

INDEX

For Product Safety Concerns and Information please contact our EU
representative GPSR@taylorandfrancis.com
Taylor & Francis Verlag GmbH, Kaufingerstraße 24, 80331 München, Germany

www.ingramcontent.com/pod-product-compliance
Lightning Source LLC
Chambersburg PA
CBHW070401270326
41926CB00014B/2653